ILLUSTRATED CASE HISTORIES

Gastroenterology

Dr Anthony I. Morris
MSc, MD, FRCP
Consultant Physician and Gastroenterologist
Royal Liverpool University Hospital
Liverpool

Dr John Y. Yiannakou
MBChB, MRCP
Registrar in Gastroenterology
Royal Liverpool University Hospital
Liverpool

Mosby-Wolfe

London Baltimore Bogotá Boston Buenos Aires Caracas Carlsbad, CA Chicago Madrid Mexico City Milan Naples, FL
New York Philadelphia St. Louis Sydney Tokyo Toronto Wiesbaden

Project Manager: Anton Lawrencepulle

Developmental Editor: Jennifer Prast

Cover Design: Pete Wilder

Illustration: Lynda Payne

Production: Michael Heath

Index: Jill Halliday

Publisher: Richard Furn

Published in 1994 by Mosby-Wolfe, an imprint of Times Mirror International Publishers Limited

Printed by Grafos S.A. Arte sobre papel, Barcelona, Spain.

ISBN 0 7234 1889 6

For full details of all Times Mirror International Publishers Limited titles, please write to Times Mirror International Publishers Limited, Lynton House, 7–12 Tavistock Square, London WC1H 9LB, England.

A CIP catalogue record for this book is available from the British Library.

Library of Congress Cataloging-in-Publication Data applied for.

Warning

The doses of pharmaceutical products given in this book are a guide only. Although every effort is made to be accurate, the authors and publishers cannot be held responsible for the accuracy of these dosages. It is recommended that the reader, if in any doubt, checks in the latest editions of publications such as the *British National Formulary*, *Martindale's Extra Pharmacopoeia* or *MIMS* (*Monthly Index of Medical Specialities*).

Contents

Preface

Each case history is presented as a challenge for the reader to formulate his/her own diagnostic and management plan, with the answers immediately following. We have been didactic where appropriate, but local practice varies enormously with geographical differences in the prevalence of pathogens and their sensitivity to antimicrobials, local or national prescribing policies and mere fashion. The case histories are suitable for postgraduate students to read alone or for discussion in group tutorials. We anticipate that one of the major challenges in either situation will be to identify areas in which local practice differs from our own answers, and to identify the reasons for this. We have tried to highlight the main points relevant to each case, and hope that these will stimulate the reader to enquire after further detail in more comprehensive textbooks or current journals.

To simplify the case histories, the majority of the common haematological and biochemical investigations have been abbreviated and presented in a stylised format. Where relevant, we have emphasised the importance of community control of infections, including timely notification. In the United Kingdom the term 'public health authorities' in the text means the local consultant in public health medicine or consultant in communicable disease control. We have used the more generic term in recognition that the appropriate statutory authority will vary in other countries.

Acknowledgements

We would like to thank all our colleagues who have helped to provide some of the illustrations for this book. Particular thanks are due to Dr N J E Wilson and Dr J Nash for their help with the histopathology. Other colleagues who provided many of the radiographic, nuclear medicine scans and other pictures are Dr C J Garvey, Dr R D Edwards, Dr P C Rowlands, Dr J F M Meaney, Dr G T Abbott, Dr M Critchley, Mr J S Brown, Dr J A Ashworth, Mr G J Poston, Mrs T Norris, Dr N Laique and Dr J Menon. We would also like to thank Sister Cottrell and the nursing staff of the Royal Liverpool University Hospital Gasstroenterology Unit for their help, advice and patience in obtaining the endoscopic pictures.

We gratefully acknowledge advice and support from Dr I T Gilmore and Dr J M Rhodes.

Dedication

To Sheila, Daniel and David for their patience, help and support. A.I.M.

To my Parents. J.Y.Y.

Case 1

Weight loss and dysphagia

A 60-year-old lady was admitted with a 3-month history of progressive weight loss of 2 stones and increasing dysphagia for solids. Before admission she had started to vomit after everything she ate or drank. She had no other symptoms and smoked 15 cigarettes per day. Her mother had died, at the age of 56, from carcinoma of the bronchus. On examination she was very anxious and had clearly lost weight.

Investigations

Haematology and Biochemistry chart on page 6; Radiology, see **1** and **2**; Endoscopy, see **3**.

Questions

1 What abnormalities are seen on the x-rays?
2 What is the differential diagnosis?
3 What further investigations are required?
4 What forms of treatment are available?

1

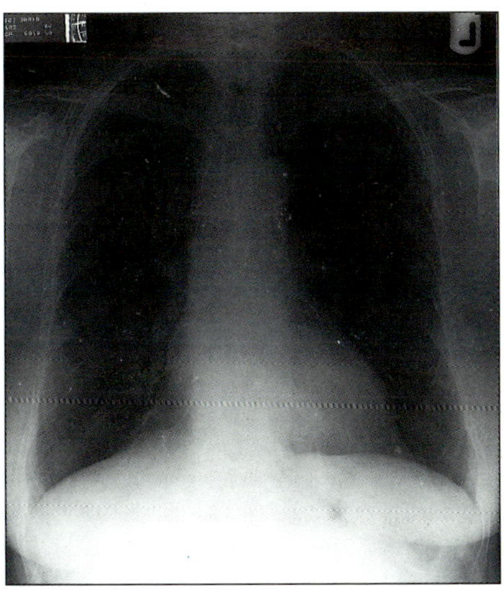

2

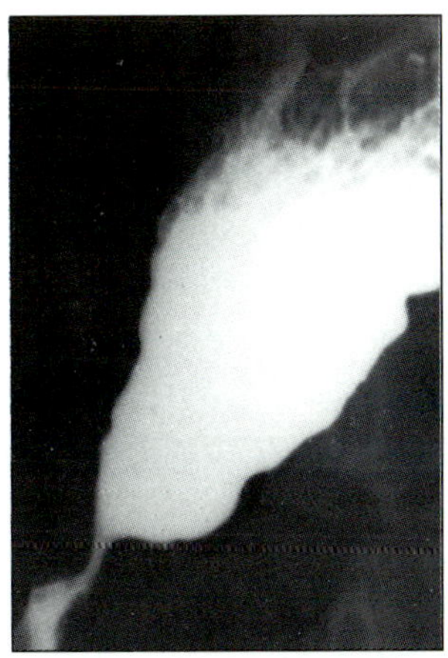

3

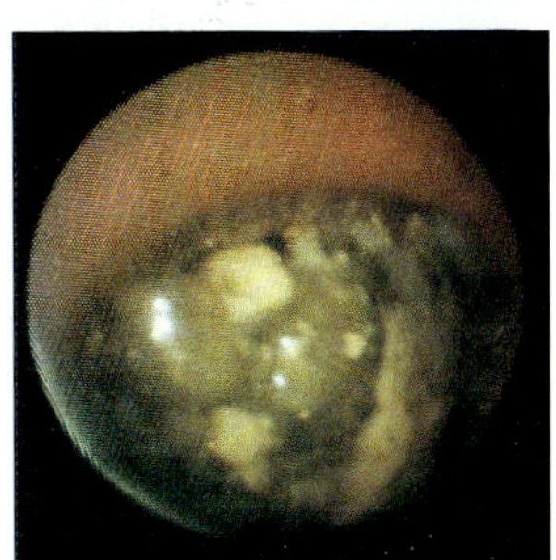

1 Chest x-ray.
2 Barium swallow.
3 Endoscopic view of the oesophagus.

		Normal Range			Normal Range
Hb	12.8	11.5–16 **g/dl**	**MCHC**	33.7	33–36 **g/dl**
Hct	36	33–47 **%**	**Platelets**	254	50–400/ **10^9/l**
MCV	82	80–100 **fl**	**WCC**	8.0	3.5–11 / **10^9/l**
MCH	28	28–33 **pg**	**ESR**	28	< 20 **mm/hr**
Sodium	140	135–145**mmol/l**	**Blood sugar**	6.5	3.5–7.2 **mmol/**
Potassium	3.4	3.5–5.0 **mmol/l**	**Bilirubin**	13	2–17 **mmol/l**
Chloride	98	95–105 **mmol/l**	**Alk. Phos.**	118	35–125 **U/l**
Bicarbonate	32	20–30 **mmol/l**	**ALT**	21	0–35 **U/l**
Urea	8.4	2.5–7.0 **mmol/l**	**GGT**	30	0–35 **U/l**
Creatinine	142	50–150 **mmol/l**	**Albumin**	38	36–52 **g/l**
Phosphate	1.06	0.7–1.4 **mmol/l**	**Globulin**	26	22–32 **g/l**
Calcium	2.43	2.2–2.6 **mmol/l**	**CRP**	6	< 5**mg/l**

Answers and discussion

1 The barium swallow (**2**) shows a tapered narrowing at the lower end of the oesophagus with hold-up of the column of barium. There is no mucosal ulceration. The chest x-ray is normal (**1**).
2 The differential diagnosis must include carcinoma of the oesophagus/cardia, a benign peptic stricture and either achalasia of the oesophagus or pseudoachalasia. In certain parts of the world Chagas' disease would have to be considered.
3 The endoscopy (**3**) shows a fluid and debris filled oesophagus that would need to be repeated after aspiration of the oesophagus through a nasogastric tube, or by means of an endoscope with a large diameter suction channel. The lower end of the oesophagus appeared normal (**4**), and opened up with minimal pressure. It is then essential to examine the stomach most carefully, and particularly the area of the cardia from below (**5**) to ensure there is no malignant infiltration causing pseudoachalasia. The use of endoscopic ultrasound to delineate the layers of the oesophageal wall is particularly helpful, albeit not widely available. Figure **6** shows the ultrasound scanner at the end of the oblique viewing gastroscope, while **7a–b** demonstrate the normal layers seen with this equipment. The most important confirmatory test for achalasia is an oesophageal motility study; **8a–b** demonstrate this patient's motility study. It shows that the sphincter is of high pressure, and that it does not relax on swallowing. The other findings were of lack of normally conducted peristaltic pressure waves down the oesophagus and the presence of many synchronous multiphasic pressure waves induced by swallowing.

4

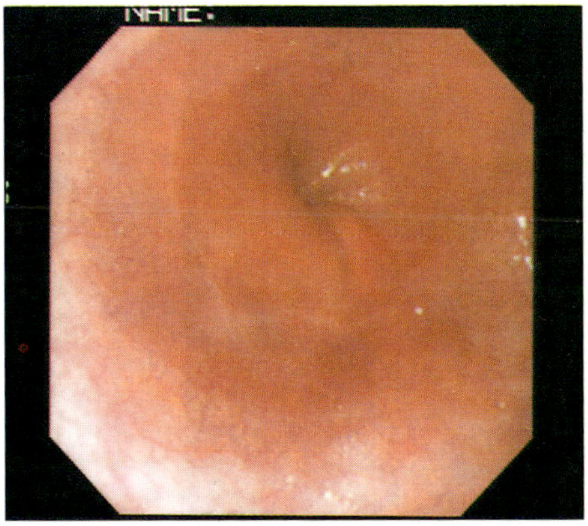

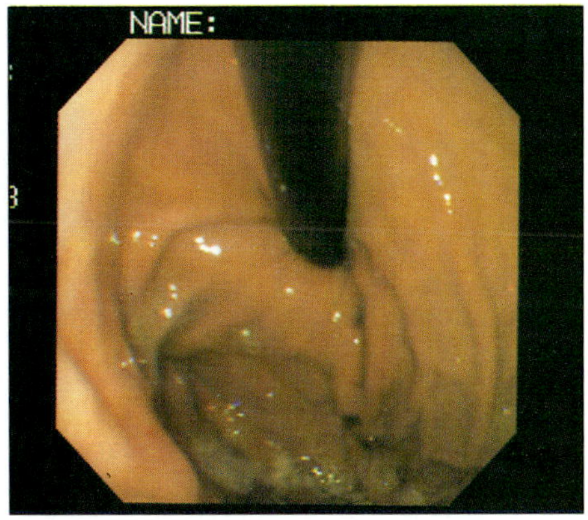

5

4 Normal lower oesophagus. Note squamocolumnar junction.

5 Examination of cardia with retroflexed scope.

6a

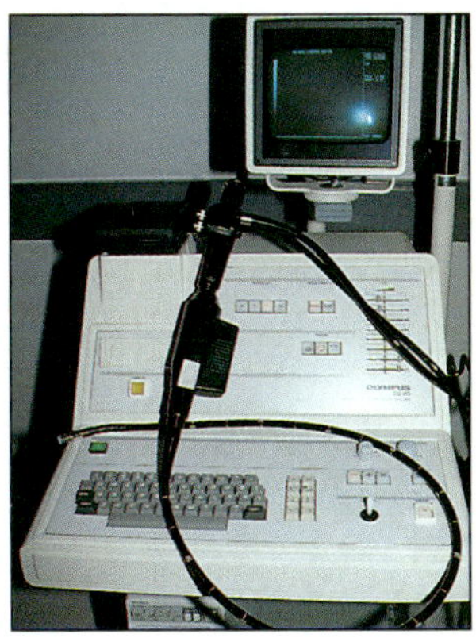

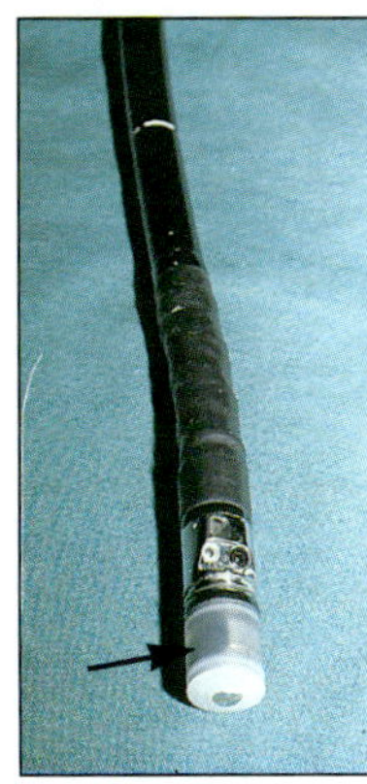

6b

6a Endoscope and scanner.
6b Ultrasound probe (arrow) at end of sideviewing endoscope.

7a

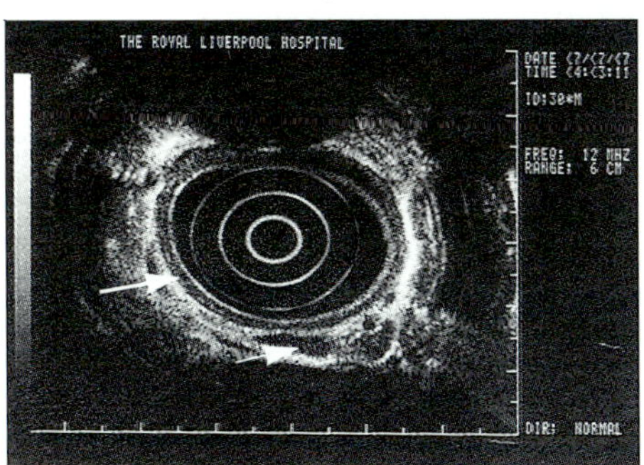

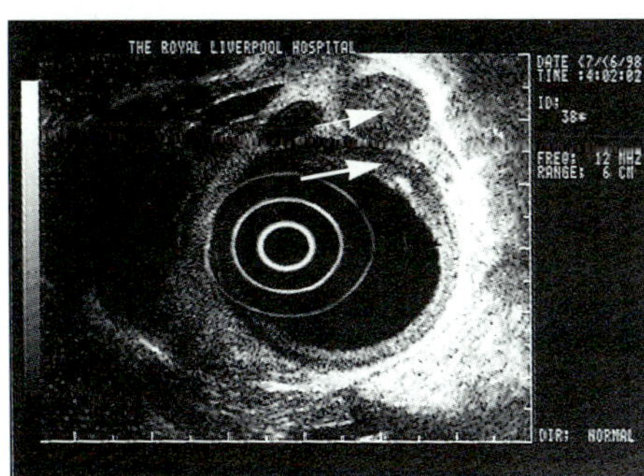

7b

7 a and **b** Endoscopic ultrasound of lower oesophagus. **a**) Normal appearance showing five-layered mucosa (thick arrow) and normal lymph nodes (thin arrow). **b**) An infiltrating mucosal carcinoma producing loss of five-layered structure and expansion of mucosal layer (thick arrow). The lymph nodes (thin arrow) are expanded and abnormal.

8a

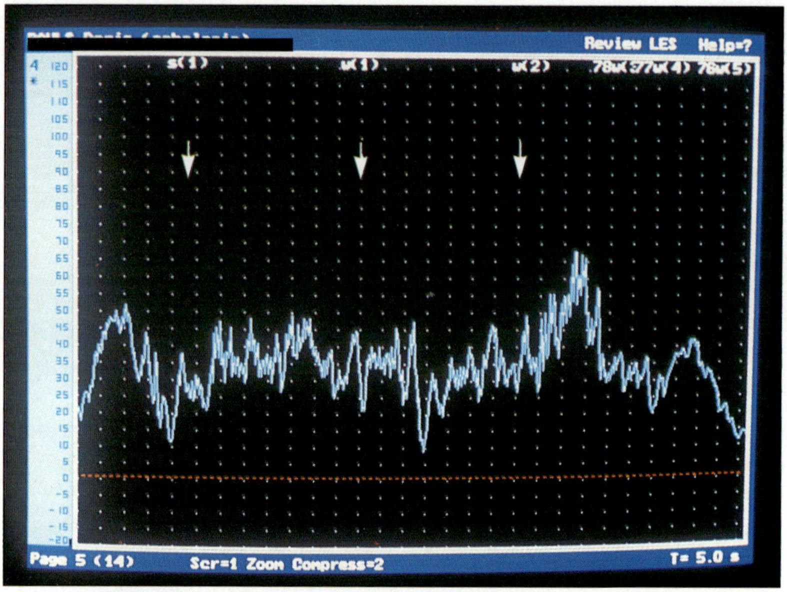

8b

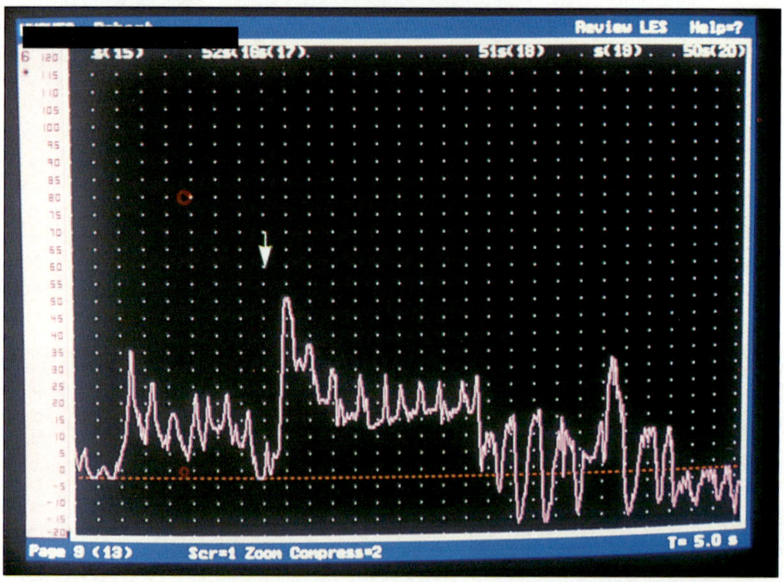

8 Oesophageal manometry: **a**) Achalasia, **b**) Normal. The tracings show the pressure at the lower oesophageal sphincter. In the normal study the pressure falls to equalibrate with intragastric pressure with each swallow.The tracing from the patient shows sustained high pressure.

4 Once the diagnosis has been established, three forms of treatment are available. For patients with the more classical, milder, intermittent symptoms, a trial of a smooth muscle relaxing drug such as isosorbide mononitrate, or the calcium channel antagonist, nifedipine, can sometimes control the patients' symptoms well. In those patients who derive no benefit, or who are symptomatically severe, as in this case, the choice lies between Pneumatic Balloon Dilatation and surgery in the form of a Heller's myotomy.

In many countries initial treatment is with balloon dilatation. Figure **9** is one example of such a dilating system. This is usually performed under x-ray control and the oesophagus dilated to 3–3.5 cm.

9

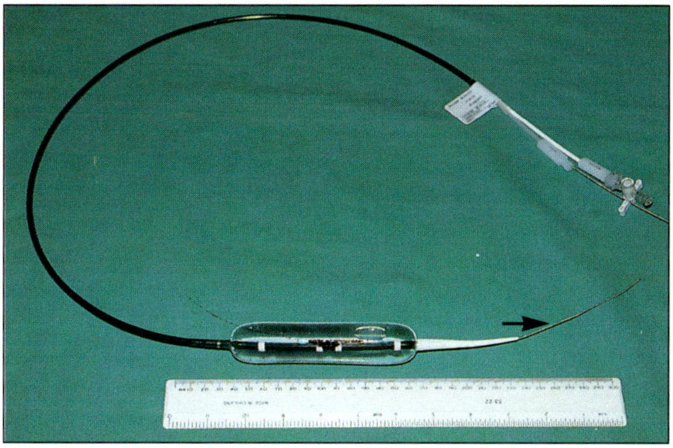

9 The balloon is placed over a guidewire (arrow) and is filled with contrast medium so that it can be seen on fluorsocopy.

Many gastroenterologists would attempt one or two such dilatations before referring the patient for myotomy. With the advent of minimally invasive surgery, laparoscopic myotomy may well replace open surgery in experienced hands. All such operations carry the risk of rendering the lower oesophageal sphincter totally incompetent and thus allowing the development of significant oesophageal reflux. To prevent this some surgeons combine the Heller's myotomy with an anti-reflux procedure at the same time.

Clinical progress

This patient had a single pneumatic balloon dilatation to 3.0 cm. Following this her swallowing returned to normal and she regained all the lost weight in 8 weeks. Although the usual history for a patient with achalasia is that of intermittent dysphagia for liquids and solids, some patients relate a history much more like that of malignant stricture, as in this case. The negative endoscopic ultrasound examination and subsequent follow-up have excluded pseudoachalasia.

Case 2

Cough induced by drinking

A 67-year-old man presented with a 2-month history of progressive dysphagia for solids associated with weight loss of 7 kg over the same period. In the 3 weeks immediately before being seen in the outpatient department he noted that whenever he drank fluids he would get a spasm of coughing. These attacks of coughing were so severe that by admission he could tolerate nil by mouth. He was a heavy smoker, and consumed alcohol in moderation. On examination the only important abnormality was a firm liver 6 cm below the costal margin.

Investigations

Haematology and Biochemistry chart on page 11; Chest x-ray, see **1;** Niopam swallow, see **2**; Ultrasound scan of liver, see **3**; Endoscopy, see **4**.

Questions

1 What does the history suggest is wrong with this patient?
2 What do the x-rays and ultrasound scan show?
3 What further investigation is indicated?
4 What treatment is available for this patient?

1

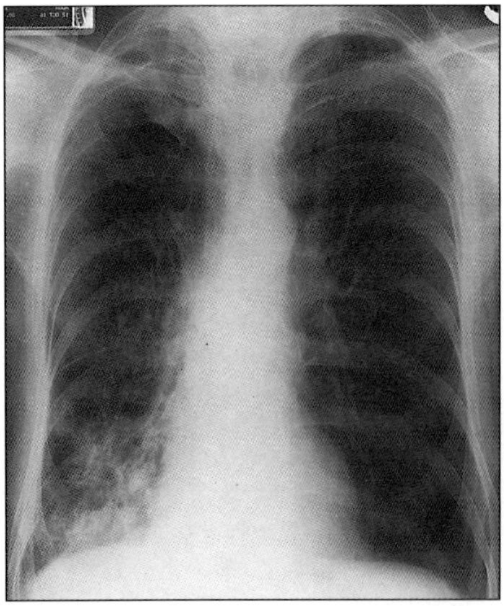

1 Chest x-ray.

2

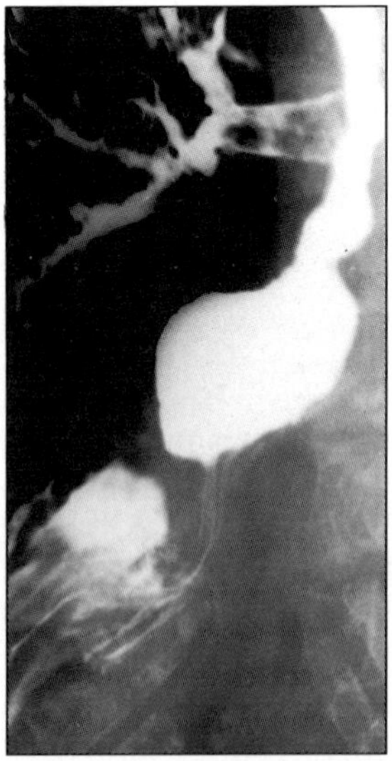

2 Niopam swallow.

		Normal Range			Normal Range
Hb	9.6	12.5–18 **g/dl**	**MCHC**	31.0	33–36 **g/dl**
Hct	32.3	33–47 **%**	**Platelets**	170	150–400/ **10^9/l**
MCV	67.2	80100 **fl**	**WCC**	10.2	3.5–11 / **10^9/l**
MCH	22.6	28–33 **pg**	**ESR**	52	< 5 **mm/hr**
Sodium	147	135–145 **mmol/l**	**Blood sugar**	5.5	3.5–7.2 **mmol/l**
Potassium	4.6	3.5–5.0 **mmol/l**	**Bilirubin**	32	2–17 **mmol/l**
Chloride	100	95–105 **mmol/l**	**Alk. Phos.**	1260	35–125 **U/l**
Bicarbonate	26	20–30 **mmol/l**	**ALT**	65	0–35 **U/l**
Urea	10.8	2.5–7.0 **mmol/l**	**GGT**	85	0–35 **U/l**
Creatinine	148	50–150 **mmol/l**	**Albumin**	39	36–52 **g/l**
Phosphate	1.21	0.7–1.4 **mmol/l**	**Globulin**	22	22–32 **g/l**
Calcium	2.46	2.2–2.6 **mmol/l**	**CRP**	13	< 5 **mg/l**

3

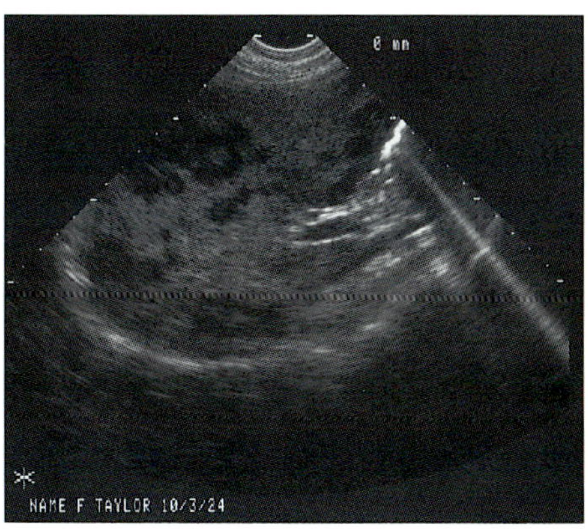

3 Ultrasound scan of liver.

4

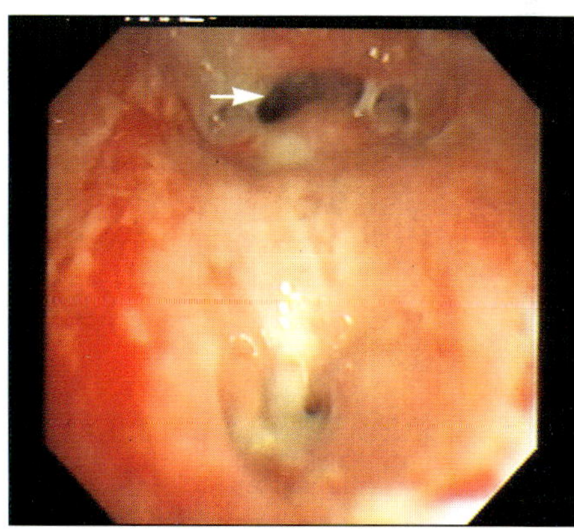

4 Endoscopy.

Answers and discussion

1 The history suggests aspiration of the ingested fluids. Without the preceding history of the progressive dysphagia this should raise the possibility of a neuromuscular problem affecting the pharynx. A bulbar or pseudobulbar palsy might cause such symptoms such as could be seen with motor neurone disease.The history of preceding dysphagia raises two possibilities. If there was a benign stricture as the cause of the dysphagia then aspiration overflow would give this symptom, however if the underlying pathology was a malignancy then this history should suggest a Tracheo-Oesophageal Fistula.

2 The chest x-ray (**1**) shows basal shadowing on the right consistent with aspiration changes. The Niopam swallow (**2**) shows a Tracheo-Oesophageal Fistula with a malignant stricture in the oesophagus. The ultrasound scan (**3**) shows multiple low density areas in the liver consistent with metastases.

3 The only other investigation of relevance to this patient's management is a biopsy of the malignant stricture seen on endoscopy. Biopsy is important to ascertain what cellular type of tumour was present. In this case biopsy showed a squamous-cell carcinoma (**5**). Unusually in this case it was possible to actually see the fistulous connection (**4** arrow). Frequently no opening is seen, particularly in long, exophytic, friable tumours, and the clue to the presence of a fistula is obtained from the history later to be confirmed by contrast radiology. If a fistula is being sought then it is normal to use contrast media other than barium which is very irritant to the bronchial tree.

Figure **6** shows a benign fistula to the right lower lobe in a patient with long-standing oesophageal reflux and a stricture. There was no reliable history despite the size of the fistula as the patient was schizophrenic.

4 There are two methods of treating a malignant tracheo-oesophageal fistula. Both unfortunately are palliative as surgical resection for such a malignant fistula is rarely undertaken on the grounds of difficulty and incurability. The main

5

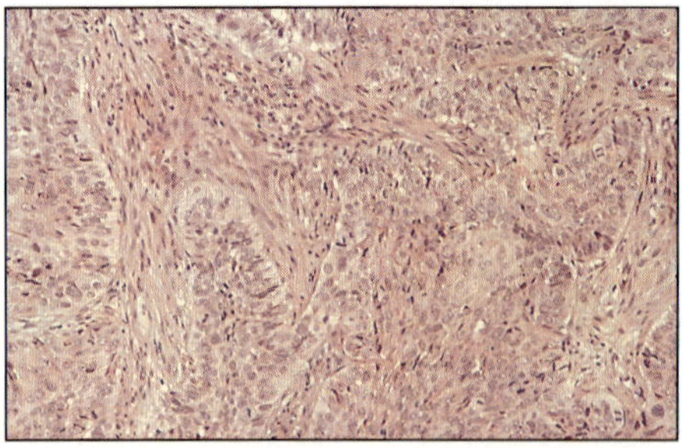

5 Oesophageal biopsy showing disorganised cell structure and keratinisation typical of a squamous carcinoma.

6

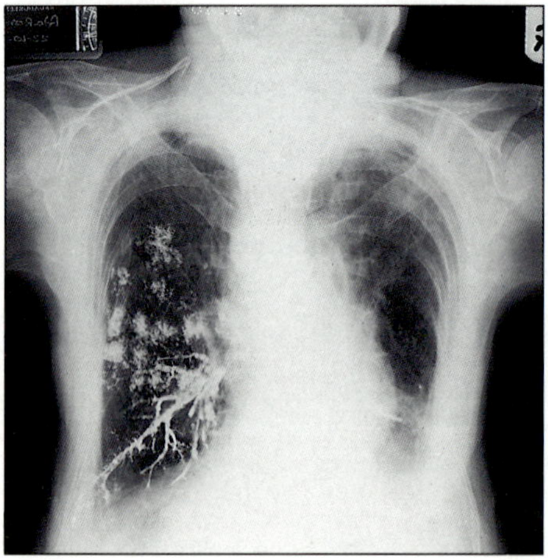

6 Benign fistula in right lobe.

method of treatment involves the placement of a prosthetic tube (**7a–c**) through the stricture (**8**) to stent the malignancy and at the same time obturate the fistulous opening. After dilatation of the stricture to an adequate size (about 18 mm) the prosthetic tube can be pushed through under radiological control. Either a plain tube can be used or if available a cuffed tube can be used. In this there is a cuff of foam which is deflated prior to placement and subsequently allowed to inflate to block the fistula gently. The placement of a prosthetic tube carries a 10% perforation rate. Figures **7a–c** show a selection of prosthetic tubes.

7a

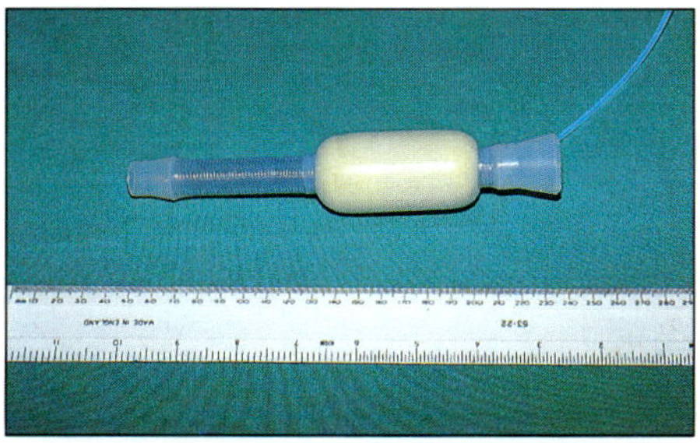

7b

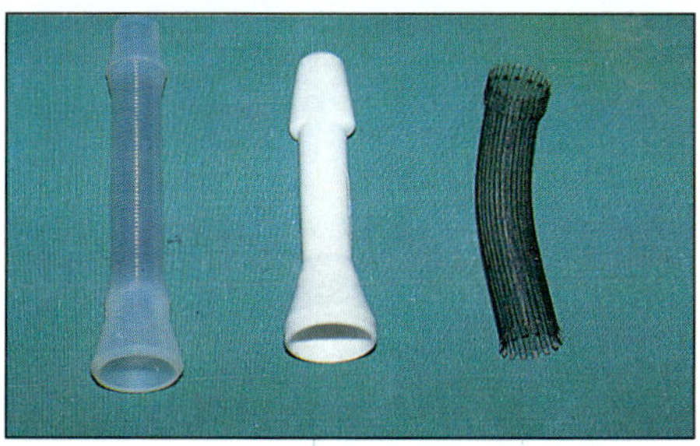

7c

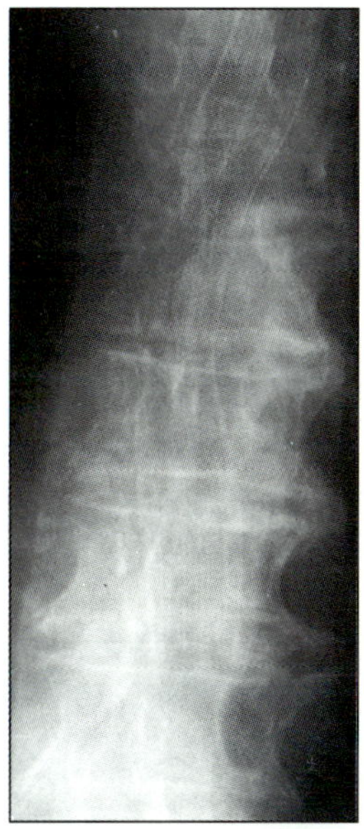

7 Oesophageal stents: **a**) Inflated cuffed prosthesis; **b**) Selection of prosthesis including an expanding-metal wall stent (right). **c**) Expanding-metal wall stent in a patient with oesophageal carcinoma.

8

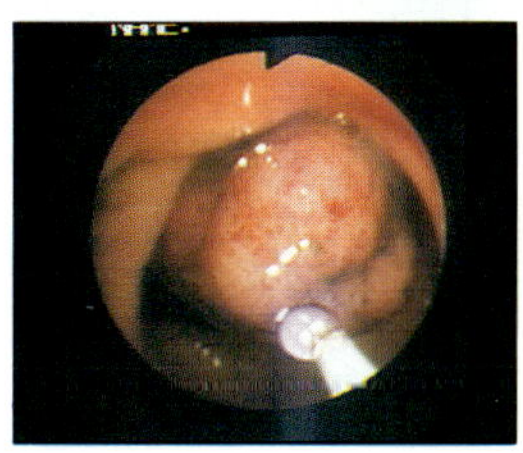

8 Tumour being lasered.

The alternative form of treatment is to perform a Percutaneous Endoscopic Gastrostomy to permit feeding without the risk of aspiration. This option is infrequently used as it does not effectively palliate the aspiration of swallowed saliva.

Clinical progress

The patient went on to have a cuffed prosthetic tube inserted. He had no further problems with aspiration and was able to swallow all liquids and semi-solids for the rest of his life. He died of disseminated malignancy 6 weeks later. Contraindications to surgical resection of oesophageal malignancy include in addition to fistulation into the bronchial tree, evidence of metastases, a long tumour, and an unfit patient.

Case 3

Distressing chest pain at rest

A 48-year-old company director developed central chest pain radiating down his left arm while driving his car. He had felt similar, but milder pain on several preceding occasions usually when under stress. He had awoken with pain of a similar nature in the middle of the night on several occasions in the past few weeks. He smoked 25 cigarettes per day and both parents had died in their 50s of myocardial infarction. He drove straight to the local hospital, where on examination, apart from a tachycardia and anxiety, there were no abnormal physical signs.

Investigations

Haematology and Biochemistry chart on page 15. Serial cardiac enzymes – Normal x 3; Electrocardiogram – Normal x 3; Barium swallow, see **1**; Endoscopy, see **2**. Chest x-ray normal.

Questions

1 What abnormality is seen on the barium swallow?
2 What does the endoscopy show?
3 What further investigations are required?
4 What does the 24 hour pH study demonstrate?
5 What treatments are available for this problem?

1

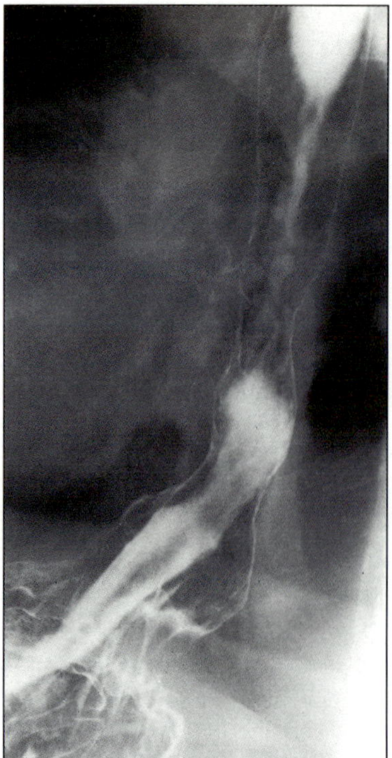

1 Barium swallow.

2

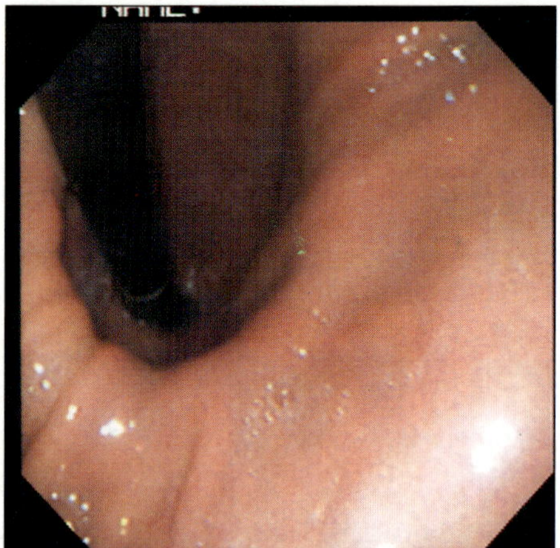

2 Retroflexed view of cardia.

		Normal Range			Normal Range
Hb	16.9	12.5–18 **g/dl**	**MCHC**	34.4	33–36 **g/dl**
Hct	49.2	33–47 **%**	**Platelets**	212	150–400/ **10^9/l**
MCV	89.9	80–100 **fl**	**WCC**	10.6	3.5–11 **/ 10^9/l**
MCH	31.0	28–33 **pg**	**ESR**	2	< 5 **mm/hr**
Sodium	143	135–145 **mmol/l**	**Blood sugar**	5.4	3.5–7 **mmol/l**
Potassium	4.0	3.5–5.0 **mmol/l**	**Bilirubin**	5	2–17 **mmol/l**
Chloride	106	95–105 **mmol/l**	**Alk. Phos.**	107	35–125 **U/l**
Bicarbonate	28	20–30 **mmol/l**	**ALT**	18	0–35 **U/l**
Urea	4.6	2.5–7.0 **mmol/l**	**GGT**	22	0–35 **U/l**
Creatinine	88	50–150 **mmol/l**	**Albumin**	47	36–52 **g/l**
Phosphate	1.18	0.7–1.4 **mmol/l**	**Globulin**	25	22–32 **g/l**
Calcium	2.42	2.2–2.6 **mmol/l**	**CRP**	<5	5 **mg/l**
Creatine kinase		(1), (2) and (3)			

Answers and discussion

1 The barium swallow (**1**) shows some reflux and a small sliding hiatus hernia.
2 The endoscopy (**2**) shows a small hiatus hernia with no evidence of oesophagitis.
3 Although it is always tempting to blame chest pain and dyspeptic symptoms on a hiatus hernia, these are often coincidental findings and may not be the cause of the patient's symptoms. Even if the endoscopy had shown oesophagitis (**3** and **4**) in a patient of this age, with his family and smoking history, it would be unwise to accept a static ECG as indicating there is no ischaemic heart disease. An exercise ECG should be carried out as the first step. The summary printout of his exercise test is shown in **5**. There was no evidence of significant abnormality after adequate exercise according to the Bruce Protocol.

In the light of this information the next most likely cause for his chest pain was oesophageal. The presence of reflux demonstrated on a barium x-ray is not a reliable guide as to whether either the patient has significant reflux, or whether the reflux is the cause of his symptoms. In addition, motility abnormalities may not be seen on a standard barium examination. The patient should have an oesophageal motility study to exclude diffuse oesophageal spasm as a cause for his pain and in addition should have a 24-hour oesophageal pH recording.
4 The 24-hour recording (**6**) shows frequent episodes of reflux, taken as the time when the pH in the oesophagus is below pH4. In addition the event marker demonstrated that when he had chest pain, this corresponded to an episode of reflux (**6**). The equipment used for recording pH in the oesophagus is shown in **7**. It consists of a fine pH sensitive electrode mounted on a soft transnasal catheter, which is connected to a portable tape recorder that is worn on a belt by the patient. At the end of the recording period the tape is played back through a computer for analysis of the pH profile.

3 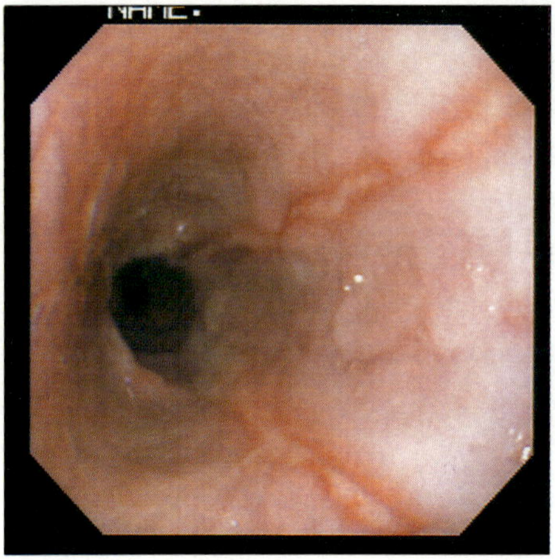

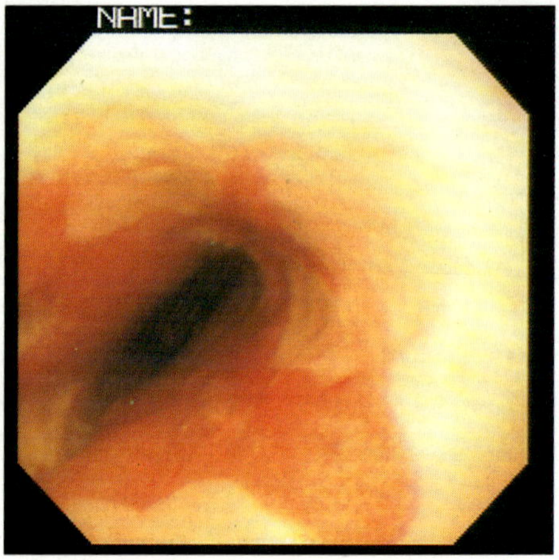 4

3 Grade II Oesophagitis. There are confluent erosions but these do not cover the whole circumference.

4 Grade III Oesophagitis. Ulceration extends around the whole circumference. The endoscope passes through easily and there is no fixed structure.

5 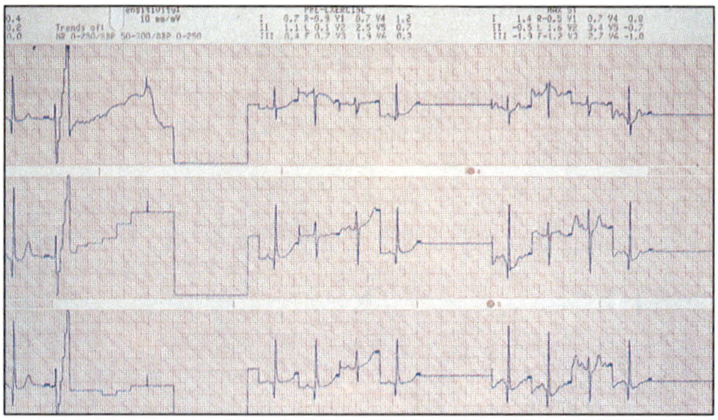

5 ECG tracing.

5 This patient had a normal exercise ECG and oesophageal manometry study as well as no evidence of oesophagitis on endoscopy. His 24-hour pH study was grossly abnormal showing significant reflux. Management of oesophageal reflux involves consideration of modification of the patient's lifestyle, the use of drugs to reduce or prevent the extent of reflux or the consideration of surgery.

Smoking is well known to relax the lower oesophageal sphincter and thus the patient should be encouraged to give up smoking. Elevation of the head of the bed by 15 cm reduces reflux, and is one of of the only physical methods that has been shown to heal oesophagitis. Taking smaller meals and avoiding food or fluids for several hours before going to bed all produce some symptomatic relief.

The mainstay of medical therapy after symptomatic treatment with antacids involves drugs designed either to reduce gastric acid secretion such as the

6 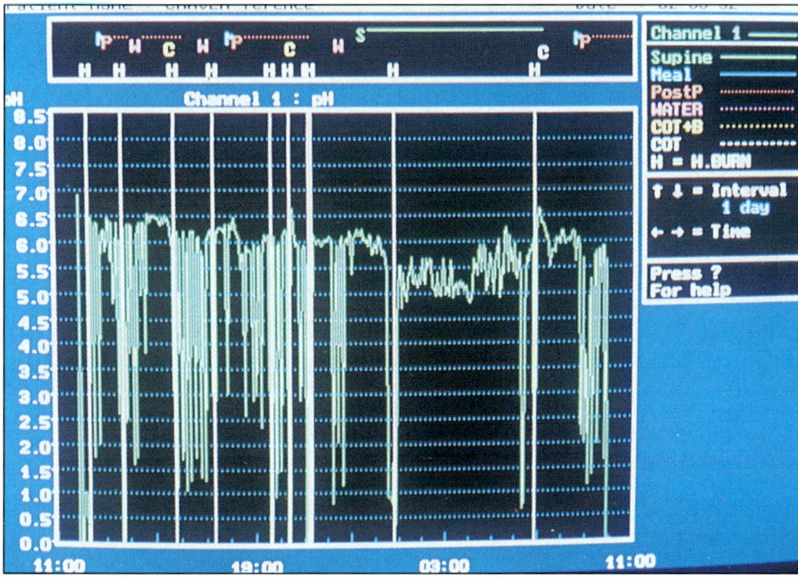

6 24-hour pH Monitoring. The frequent episodes of heartburn (H) correspond with significant drops in oesophageal pH, confirming the presence of acid reflux.

7 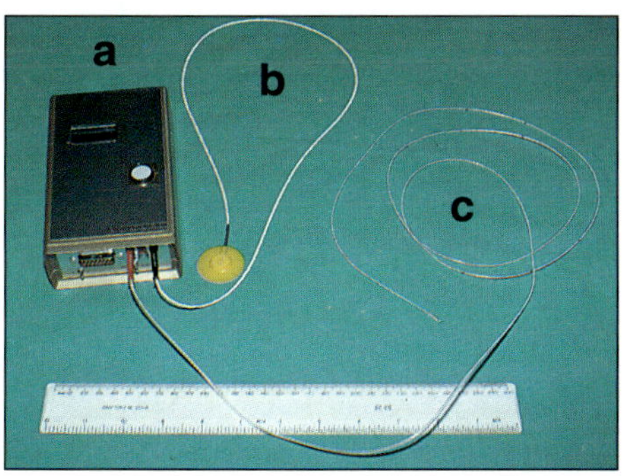

7 Equipment for pH monitoring:
a) Recording unit
b) Skin electrode
c) Naso-oesophageal probe.

Histamine H_2 Receptor Antagonists or the newer and more potent Proton Pump Inhibitors, or drugs designed to enhance gastric emptying and increase lower oesophageal sphincter pressure, such as the prokinetic agent cisapride. If drug therapy is ineffective, or the patient is unwilling to consider taking long-term drugs, then anti-reflux surgery should be considered.

Clinical progress

Initial attempts to reduce his reflux symptoms with ranitidine and cisapride failed and it was only when he was started on high-dose omeprazole that his symptoms disappeared. Whenever the dose was reduced below 40 mg/day his symptoms returned. He did not want to consider surgery as an option, even laparascopic anti- reflux surgery and is content and symptom free on omeprazole.

Case 4

Young man with jaundice

While living in a student hostel in London this 22-year-old man became anorexic and then started to feel sick and vomit. These symptoms lasted about a week and started to improve as he noticed he had become jaundiced. His urine was darker than normal and his stools became paler. Because he felt generally unwell, he returned to his parental home before he sought medical help. In his past history 2 years previously, he had developed bloody diarrhoea and investigation had shown him to have Crohn's colitis. He had been maintained on steroids and mesalazine, but whenever the steroids had been reduced he had relapsed. As a result, for the past year he had been maintained on mesalazine 800 mg t.d.s. and azathioprine 50 mg b.d. He had been off all steroids for 1 year prior to the onset of the jaundice. Investigation 9 months earlier had been normal, including Full Blood Count, CRP, Liver Function Tests.

Investigations

Haematology and Biochemistry chart on page 19; Ultrasound scans see **1a–f**.

Questions

1 What are the possible causes of his jaundice?
2 What further investigations would you arrange ?

1a

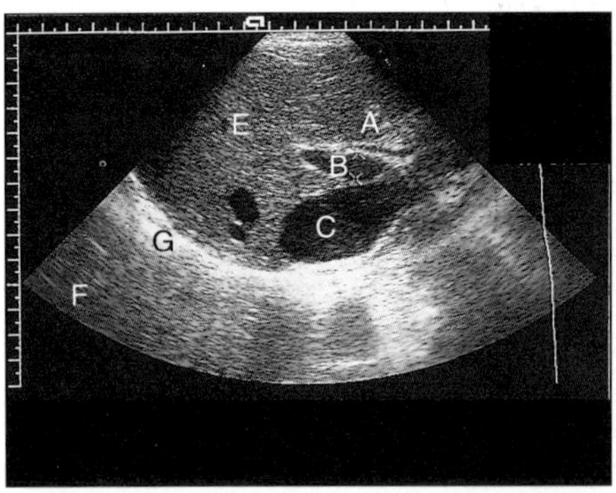

1b

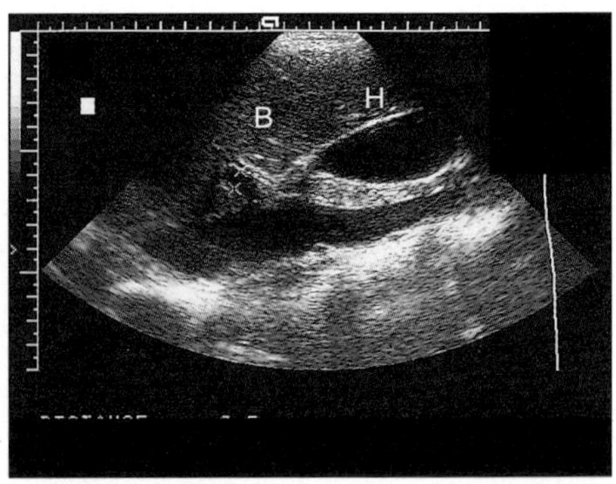

1a–1f Ultrasound scans: (see key on page 19).

1c

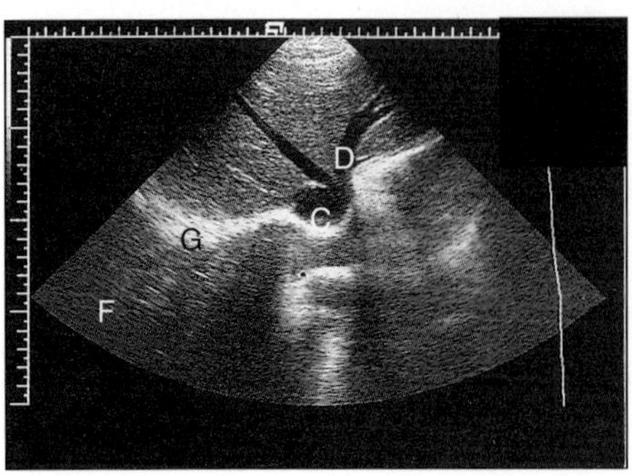

1d

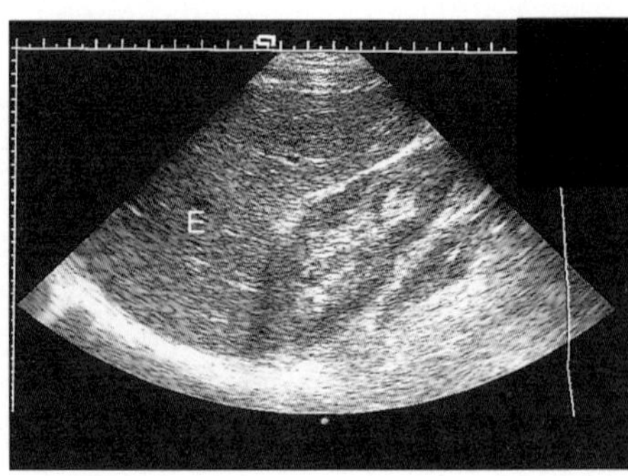

1e

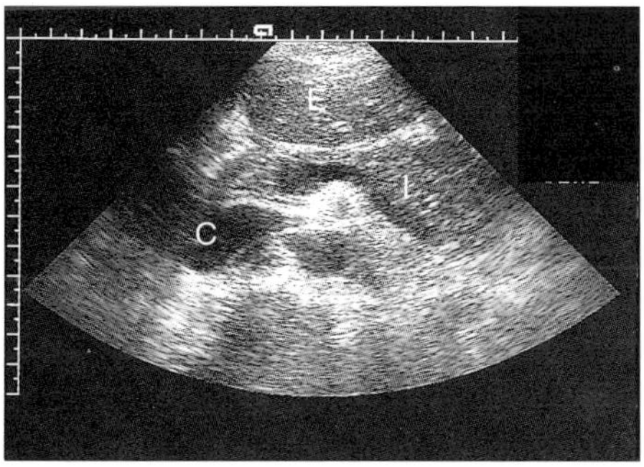

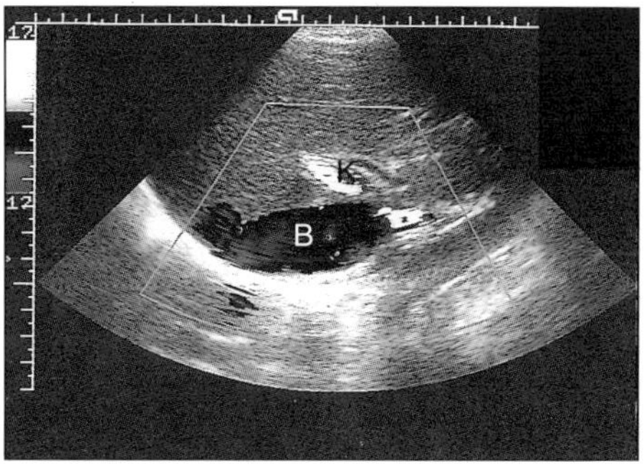

1f

Key to normal ultrasound scans

A Common duct	G Diaphragm
B Portal vein	H Gall bladder
C IVC	I Pancreas
D Hepatic veins	J Superior mesenteric artery
E Liver	K Hepatic artery
F Lung	

		Normal Range			Normal Range
Hb	12.6	12.5–18 **g/dl**	**MCHC**	35.1	33–36 **g/dl**
Hct	36.4	33–47 %	**Platelets**	246	150–400/ **10^9/l**
MCV	82.0	80–100 **fl**	**WCC**	8.4	3.5–11 **/ 10^9/l**
MCH	29.0	28–33 **pg**	**ESR**	28	< 5 **mm/hr**
Sodium	136	135–145 **mmol/l**	**Blood sugar**	3.8	3.5–7.2 **mmol/l**
Potassium	3.9	3.5–5.0 **mmol/l**	**Bilirubin**	230	2–17 **mmol/l**
Chloride	103	95–105 **mmol/l**	**Alk. Phos.**	1256	35–125 **U/l**
Bicarbonate	22	20–30 **mmol/l**	**ALT**	897	0–35 **U/l**
Urea	4.5	2.5–7.0 **mmol/l**	**GGT**	660	0–35 **U/l**
Creatinine	72	50–150 **mmol/l**	**Albumin**	32	36–52 **g/l**
Phosphate	1.33	0.7–1.4 **mmol/l**	**Globulin**	34	22–32 **g/l**
Calcium	2.18	2.2–2.6 **mmol/l**	**CRP**	5	<5 **mg/l**

Case 4

Answers and comments

1 Acute viral hepatitis (A, B or C) would be most likely, followed by other viruses, in view of the fact that he was immunosuppressed at the time. Drug-induced jaundice would also be very likely. There is an association between auto-immune chronic active hepatitis and inflammatory bowel disease, although this is more common with ulcerative colitis. Sclerosing cholangitis is another uncommon association with Crohn's disease.

2 Viral antibody studies and auto-antibodies would be the first investigations. While awaiting the results, investigation of his clotting status would be prudent. With the exception of a positive anti-nuclear antibody (1:256), all the other tests were negative and clotting was normal. There are two final investigations that are required: a liver biopsy to assess the extent of parenchymal damage and an ERCP to delineate the bile ducts to confirm or exclude sclerosing cholangitis.

Questions

3 What does the ERCP (**2**) show ?
4 What does the liver biopsy (**3**) demonstrate ?
5 What treatment would you give in the short term ?
6 What long-term treatment may be required?

2

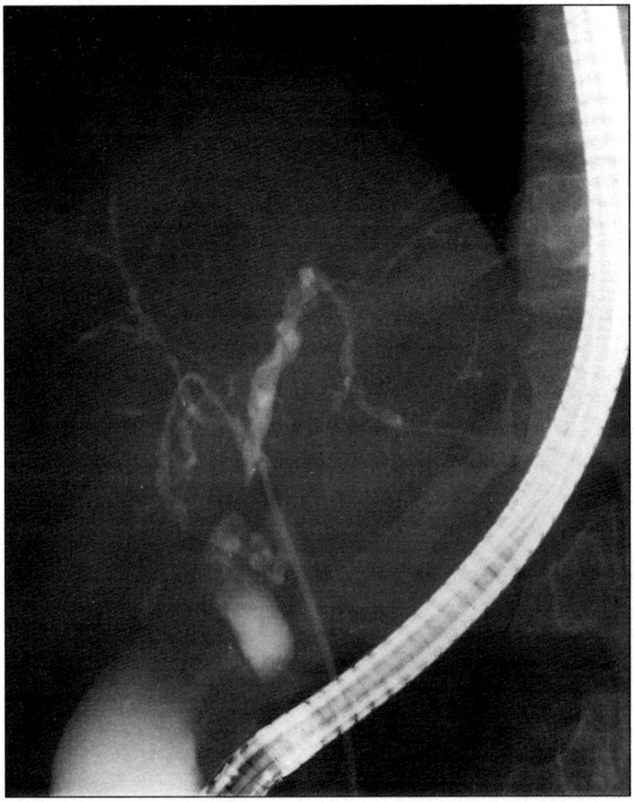

2 An ERCP of the patient.

3

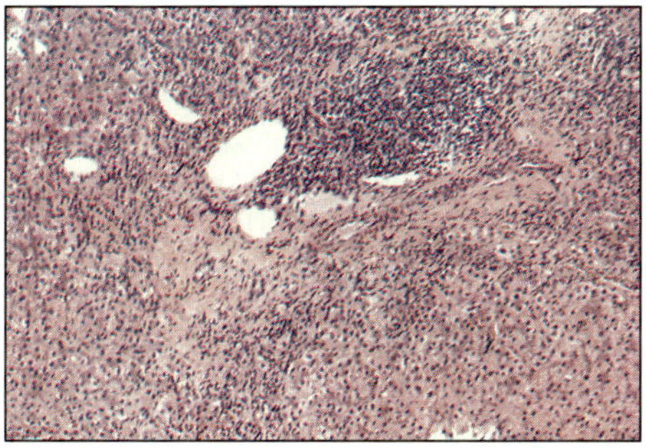

3 Liver biopsy.

Answers and comments

3 The ERCP was undertaken to delineate the bile duct and no pancreatogram was obtained. A balloon catheter was placed in the bile duct to try and distend the biliary tract. The appearances of the cholangiogram are classical for sclerosing cholangitis predominately affecting the intrahepatic ducts. There is beading and stricturing throughout the duct system.

4 The liver biopsy (**3**) shows the typical pathological features of chronic active hepatitis. There is an increase of inflammatory cells in and around the portal tract and extending into the lobules. There is some bridging necrosis and piece-meal necrosis around the limiting plate of the lobules. There is no 'onion skin' fibrosis around the bile ducts, the pathognomonic feature of sclerosing cholangitis on biopsy. A more typical biopsy is shown in **4**.

This patient thus has features of both Sclerosing cholangitis (typical ERC and disproportionately high alkaline phosphatase) and Chronic Active Hepatitis (histology, high ALT and positive ANA).

5 Initial treatment is aimed at reducing the degree of liver necrosis and inflammation. Steroids were restarted and reduced to a maintenance dose of 12.5 mg. Had there been significant extra hepatic bile duct involvement with the sclerosing cholangitis, then attempted endoscopic treatment of the strictures with balloon dilatation or stenting would have been worth considering, but as the intrahepatic ducts were all diffusely involved this was not an option.

6 Were there to be further deterioration in liver function with reduction in the patients general well-being, then liver transplantation would be worth considering. Sclerosing cholangitis is one of the commoner and well-accepted indications for transplantation.

4

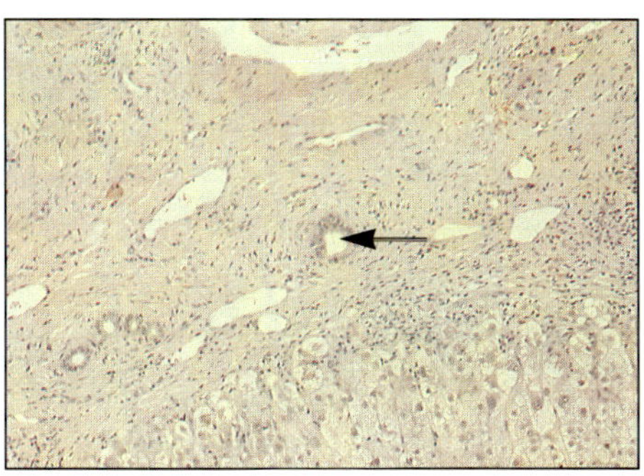

4 Liver biopsy from a patient, with sclerosing cholangitis.

Case 5

Massive gastrointestinal bleeding

An 18-year-old man was admitted after having a massive haematemesis at home. On admission he was shocked with a tachycardia of 120 and a blood pressure of 80/60. He was peripherally shut down and oliguric. He was resuscitated with plasma expanders and then blood, and received 6 units within the first few hours. At endoscopy the cause of the bleeding was easily identified (**1a** and **b**). Since 12 years of age this patient had been under follow-up because of abnormal liver function tests. Initially he had presented with jaundice and ascites, both of which had settled with conservative management.

Investigations

Haematology and Biochemistry chart on page 23. Histology, see **2** and **3**.

Questions

1 What does the endoscopy show and what are the common causes ?
2 What do the liver biopsies show and what is the main change ?
3 What are the causes of this type of liver disease in young patients?
4 What investigations are required to look for the underlying cause ?
5 How would you treat the cause of his bleeding?

1a
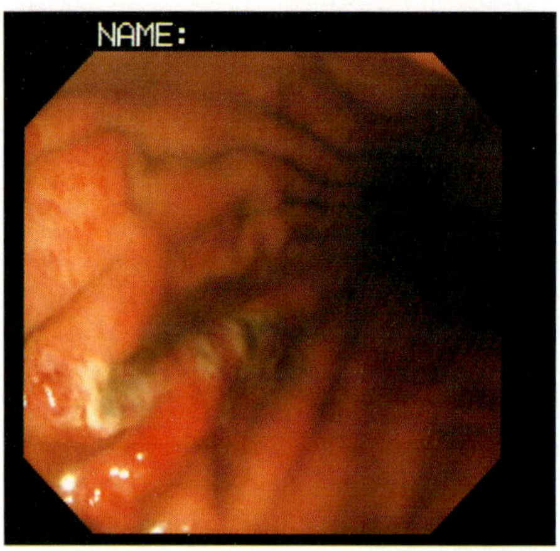

1b
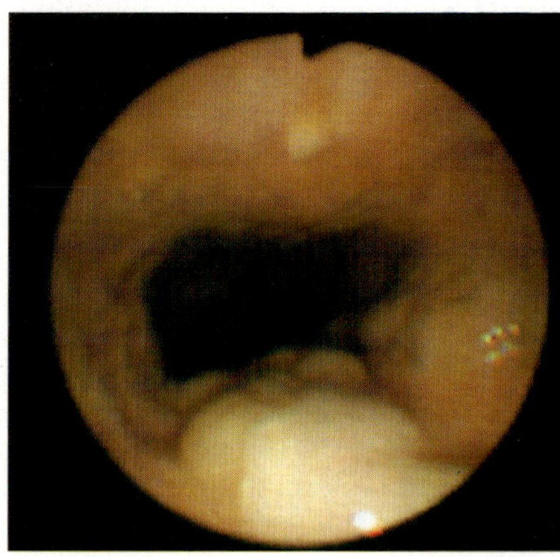

1a and **1b** Endoscopic views.
2 and **3** Histology studies of two separate liver biopsies.

2
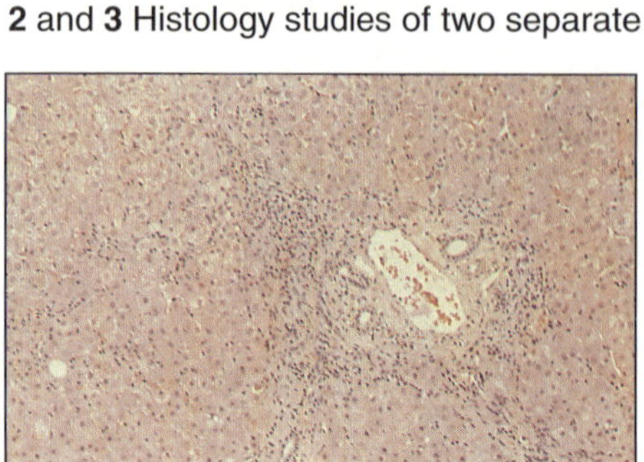

3
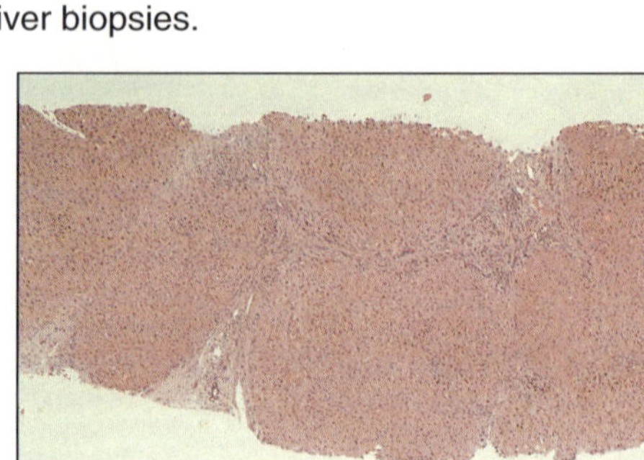

		Normal Range			Normal Range
Hb	8.6	12.5–18 **g/dl**	**MCHC**	30.0	33–36 **g/dl**
Hct	26.7	33–47 %	**Platelets**	65	150–400/ **10^9/l**
MCV	86.7	80–100 **fl**	**WCC**	12.8	3.5–11 **/ 10^9/l**
MCH	30.9	28–33 **pg**	**ESR**	18	< 10 **mm/hr**
Sodium	134	135–145 **mmol/l**	**Blood sugar**	3.8	3.5–7.2 **mmol/l**
Potassium	3.8	3.5–5.0 **mmol/l**	**Bilirubin**	89	2–17 **mmol/l**
Chloride	98	95–105 **mmol/l**	**Alk. Phos.**	187	35–125 **U/l**
Bicarbonate	22	20–30 **mmol/l**	**ALT**	236	0–35 **U/l**
Urea	6.8	2.5–7.0 **mmol/l**	**GGT**	303	0–35 **U/l**
Creatinine	60	50–150 **mmol/l**	**Albumin**	31	36–52 **g/l**
Phosphate	0.8	0.7–1.4 **mmol/l**	**Globulin**	42	22–32 **g/l**
Calcium	2.24	.2–2.6 **mmol/l**	**CRP**	7	< 5 **mg/l**
Prothrombin times		23 **sec**	**Control**		14 **sec**

Answers and comments

1 The photograph shows marked fundal gastric varices. There was only a very small oesophageal varix (**1b**). The commonest cause is secondary to cirrhosis of some type. Varices can occur with other non-cirrhotic liver diseases such as chronic active hepatitis and granulomatous hepatitis. Non-cirrhotic portal hypertension can occur as a result of portal vein thrombosis or splenic vein thrombosis or occasionally as a result of massive splenomegaly. Rarer causes include Budd–Chiari syndrome, Nodular Regenerative Hyperplasia and Idiopathic Portal Hypertension. Worldwide, one of the commonest non-cirrhotic causes for portal hypertension is Schistosomiasis.

2 The initial liver biopsy (**2**) shows changes consistent with chronic active hepatitis, with dense inflammatory infiltrate and piecemeal necrosis, whereas the subsequent liver biopsy (**3**) shows nodular regeneration, fibrosis and very little inflammatory infiltrate, the typical appearances of established cirrhosis. The nodular changes are more easily seen on the reticulin stain shown in **4a** and **b**.

3 In young patients it is particularly important to exclude genetically determined chronic liver disease. These include Wilson's Disease, cystic fibrosis, alpha 1 antitrypsin deficiency, rarely galactosaemia and haemachromatosis. The latter rarely causes cirrhosis at this age. Depending on the ethnic origin, Indian childhood cirrhosis would also have to be considered. Chronic viral hepatitis B or C would also give the same histological picture as would autoimmune chronic active hepatitis.

4 Investigation should be aimed at trying to find the underlying cause of the cirrhosis. Thus hepatitis serology for B and C virus, auto-antibodies and measurement of alpha 1 antitrypsin levels, caeruloplasmin and copper levels

4a

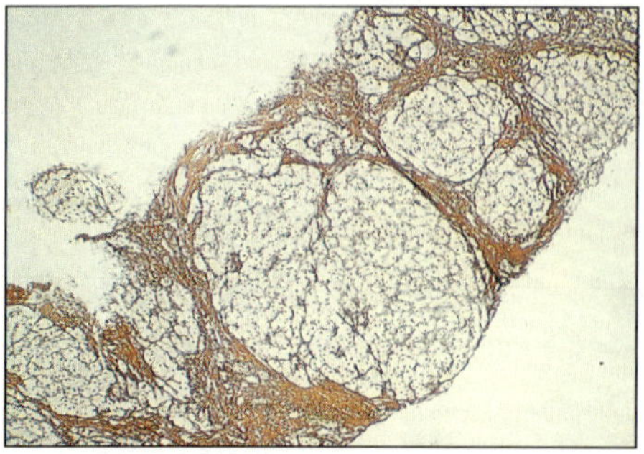

4b

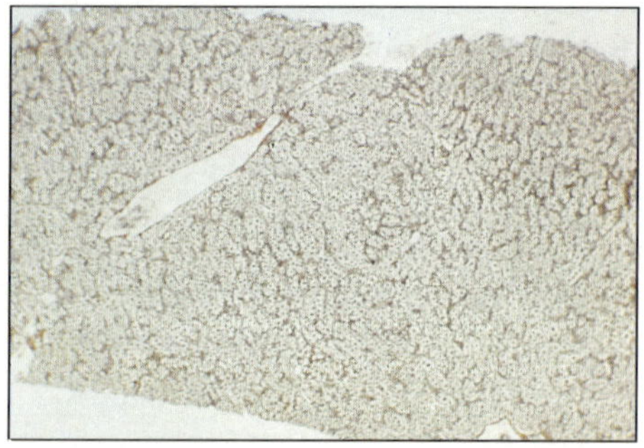

4a Reticulin stain to show nodular appearance of cirrhosis.

4b A normal one is shown for comparison.

and iron studies would be reasonable. It would be very unlikely that galactosaemia would have been missed and the patient was of caucasian stock. A slit-lamp examination for Kaiser–Fleischer rings is also helpful in excluding Wilson's Disease. This patient had been exhaustively investigated at two other centres and the cause of his chronic liver disease remains an enigma.

5 In the first instance of any patient arriving with a large gastrointestinal bleed, the most important aim is to resuscitate the patient. Once the varices have been diagnosed there are three lines of action. Which one is used depends on availability of trained staff and to a lesser extent upon equipment. The alternatives are balloon tamponade, vasoactive drugs and injection sclerotherapy. Balloon tamponade using a modified Sengstaken–Blakemore tube (**5** and **6**), is very effective at stopping bleeding but needs an experienced doctor to pass the tube to avoid complications such as airways obstruction and aspiration. The rebleeding rate is high on deflation of the balloons and it is unpleasant for the patient. The use of vasoconstrictive drugs has reduced recently, particularly the use of pitressin. It is probably the least effective of the three methods and has a high side-effect profile. Analogues of somatostatin have been claimed by some to be as effective as injection sclerotherapy, but this is debated.

The mainstay of treatment in most large centres is endoscopic injection sclerotheraphy using a suitable sclerosant suchb as polidocanol or ethanolamine oleate. The only essential equipment required is a flexible endoscopy

5

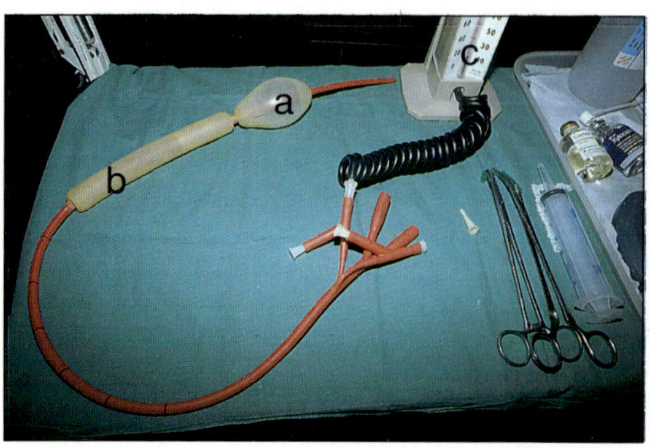

5 Minesota Tube. (a) Gastric balloon; (b) Oesophageal Balloon. (c) Manometer attached to oesophageal balloon (correct pressure 20–40 mm Hg).

6

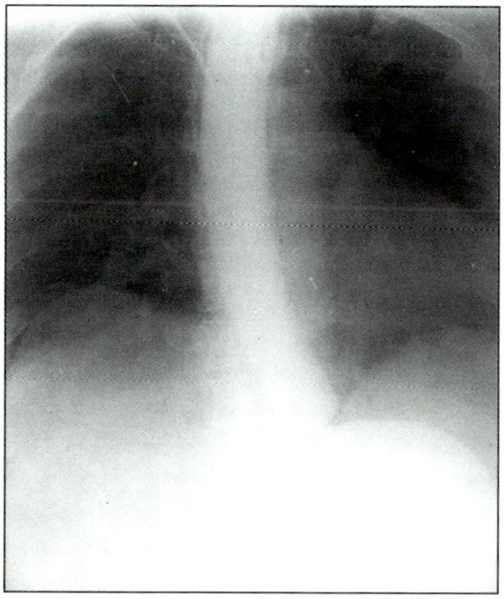

6 A modified Sengstaken–Blakemore tube being used.

7

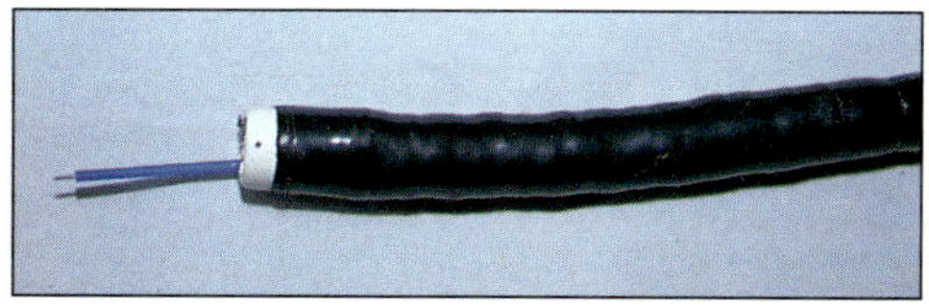

7 An injection needle at the end of a standard gastroscope.

injection needle that fits down the biopsy channel of a standard gastroscope (**7**). The use of oblique viewing or wide-channel endoscopes helps to make the technique easier by aiding access and enabling blood to be aspirated. Initial control of variceal bleeding in expert hands can be excellent and most patients then go on to further elective sclerotherapy. Until the varices are completely sclerosed the risk of further bleeding remains. It is acknowledged that fundal varices are more difficult to eradicate than oesophageal ones. If bleeding continues to be a problem, then either surgical transection of the oesophagus and/or a devascularising operation is the next step in some centres. In others a porto-systemic shunt operation would be performed for persistent variceal bleeding. More recently a new technique has become available that has the advantage of decompressing the portal system without recourse to surgery. This procedure is called Transjugular Intrahepatic Portal Systemic Stent Shunt (TIPSSS, or frequently abbreviated to TIPS).

This procedure involves the transjugular insertion of a catheter into the hepatic vein (**8**), introduction through this of a flexible needle. This is used to puncture a portal vein branch. Over a guide wire inserted through the flexible needle a catheter is placed into the portal vein and on into the superior mesenteric vein and a portagram obtained (**9**). The tract is progressively dilated between the hepatic vein and portal vein using dilating balloon catheters over a guide wire, and when the tract is large enough expanding metal wall stents are placed between the two venous systems to keep the tract patent (**10**).

The main problem of this technique is the development of encephalopathy. The shunt's size can, however, be reduced to decrease the degree of porto-systemic shunting, and in extreme cases the shunt can be occluded. Bleeding at the time of the procedure from hepatic puncture and infection around the stents are the other potential problems. The long-term performance of these shunts is still being evaluated, but one advantage of the procedure, particularly important in young patients,, is that it does not compromise future transplantation.

8

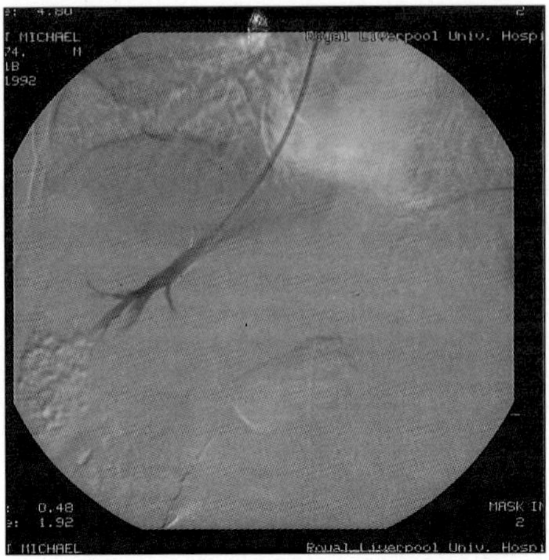

9

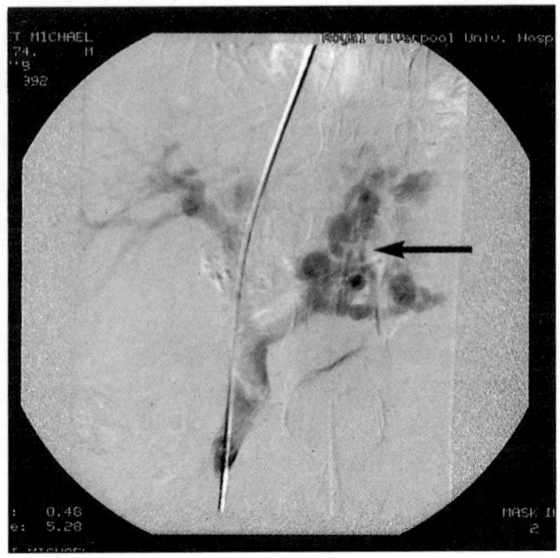

10

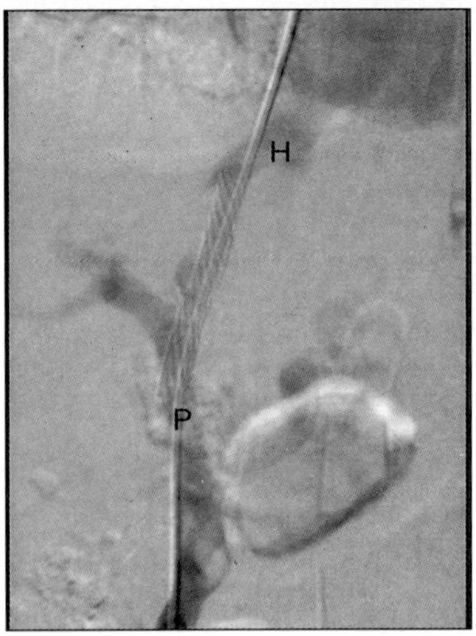

8–10 TIPS procedure.
8 Hepatic vein; **9** Portogram showing oesophago-gastric varices (arrow); **10** Placement of three Palmaz expanding-metal wall stents in the tract between the hepatic (H) and portal (P) veins.

Clinical progress

The patient had several further large bleeds over the first week despite the use of balloon tamponade and four episodes of sclerotherapy, and was transferred to a specialist centre where somatostatin and further sclerotherapy failed. He underwent a TIPS procedure 3 days before Christmas and was able to go home on Christmas day. He has not bled since and has shown no signs of encephalopathy. Six weeks after the procedure he was recatheterised to check on shunt patency and measure his portal pressure. The shunt had become occluded and was recanalised and widened to 10 mm diameter. He remains under surveillance with regular Doppler ultrasound scans.

Case 6

Abdominal swelling in a young man

This 35-year-old hotel manager was referred for an early appointment because he had developed marked abdominal swelling and peripheral oedema (**1**). He had been feeling unwell for 6 weeks with some anorexia and weight loss. His wife had noted increased jaundice for a few days. He had been under long-term surveillance since being diagnosed as having auto-immune chronic active hepatitis some 18 years previously. His liver function had normalised on prednisolone therapy and he had been well for some years on prednisolone 5 mg. His last liver biopsy performed 2 years earlier is shown in (**2**).

Investigations

Haematology and Biochemistry chart on page 28. Computed tomogram: see **3**.

1

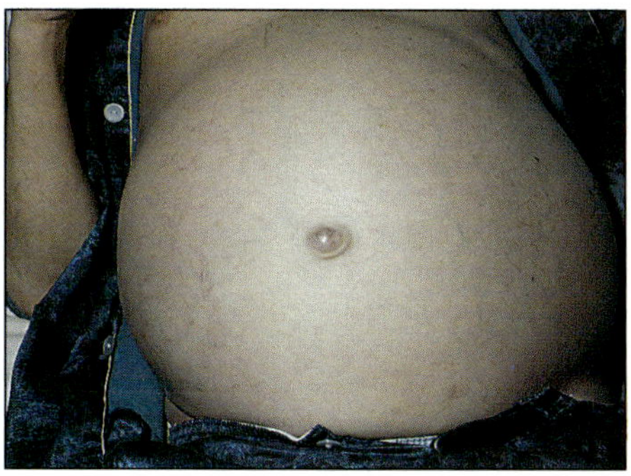

1 Abdominal distension and eversion of umbilicus secondary to ascites.

2

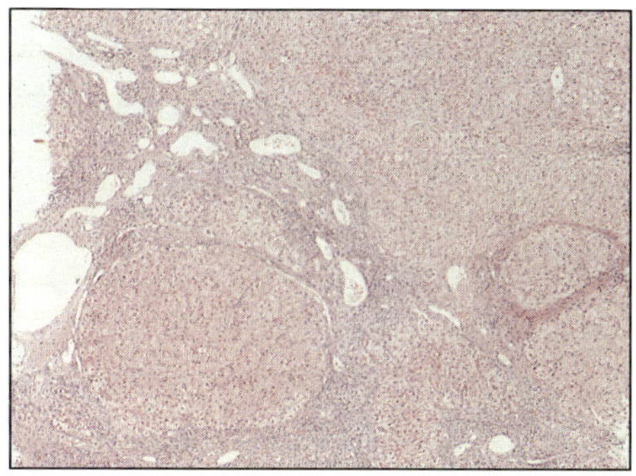

2 Liver biopsy showing fibrosis and nodular regeneration consistent with cirrhosis.

3

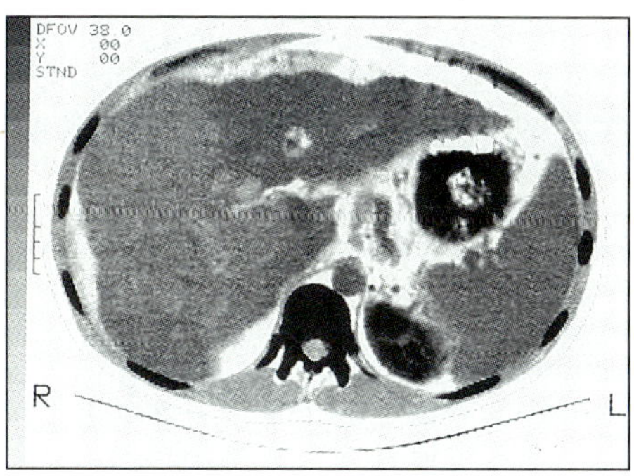

3 Computed tomogram.

Questions

1 What are the possible causes for his decompensation?
2 What other investigations should be undertaken?
3 What does the computed tomogram show?
4 What treatment options are there?

Case 6

		Normal Range			Normal Range
Hb	12.9	12.5–18 **g/dl**	**MCHC**	35.1	33–36 **g/dl**
Hct	36.1	33–47 %	**Platelets**	294	150–400/ **10^9/l**
MCV	92.7	80–100 **fl**	**WCC**	9.0	3.5–11 **/ 10^9/l**
MCH	32.2	28–33 **pg**	**ESR**	38	< 5 **mm/hr**
Sodium	137	135–145 **mmol/l**	**Blood sugar**	5.7	3.5–7.2 **mmol/l**
Potassium	3.8	3.5–5.0 **mmol/l**	**Bilirubin**	56	2–17 **mmol/l**
Chloride	100	95–105 **mmol/l**	**Alk. Phos.**	349	35–125 **U/l**
Bicarbonate	32	20–30 **mmol/l**	**ALT**	248	0–35 **U/l**
Urea	6.8	2.5–7.0 **mmol/l**	**GGT**	287	0–35 **U/l**
Creatinine	111	50–150 **mmol/l**	**Albumin**	23	36–52 **g/l**
Phosphate	0.78	0.7–1.4 **mmol/l**	**Globulin**	42	22–32 **g/l**
Calcium	2.46	2.2–2.6 **mmol/l**	**CRP**	13	< 5 **mg/l**
Prothrombin time		32 **sec**	**Control**	13 **sec**	

Answers and comments

1 There are many causes for such deterioration in a patient with chronic liver disease. The basic problem revolves around whether this is simply a deterioration in the intrinsic underlying autoimmune process or whether a complication or coincident problem has arisen. The complications that are most common are the development of a hepatocellular carcinoma or the development of spontaneous bacterial peritonitis. Spontaneous portal venous thrombosis can occur as can hepatic vein thrombosis.

2 The two most important initial investigations to be arranged are the measurement of the alpha fetoprotein level in the blood and examination of the ascitic fluid. His alpha fetoprotein was 250,000 units (< 12 U/l) and ascites microscopy and culture was negative.

3 The CT scan shows massive replacement of normal liver tissue by low-density irregular tumour, consistent with a hepatoma.

4 The outlook of a patient with a hepatoma depends upon whether it is resectable. If the tumour is resectable, then using modern technology this can be done safely and with minimal blood loss despite the presence of cirrhosis. By the use of an ultrasound dissector or high pressure water jet dissecting equipment (**4a** and **b**)specialised centres are reporting successful removal of even quite large single tumours. It is thus important to look carefully to exclude any evidence of extra hepatic spread as well as for multiple lesions within the liver.

4a 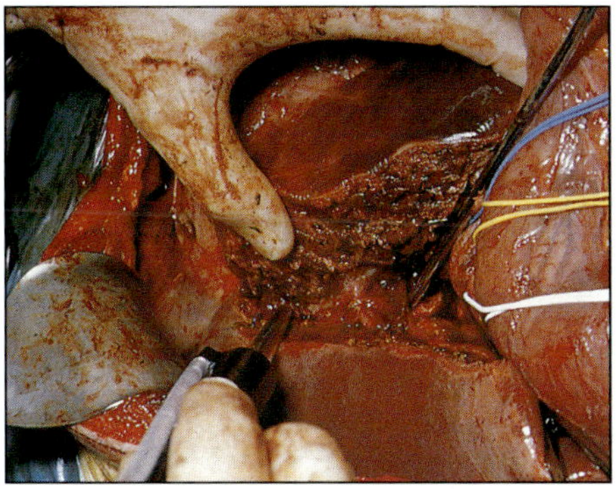 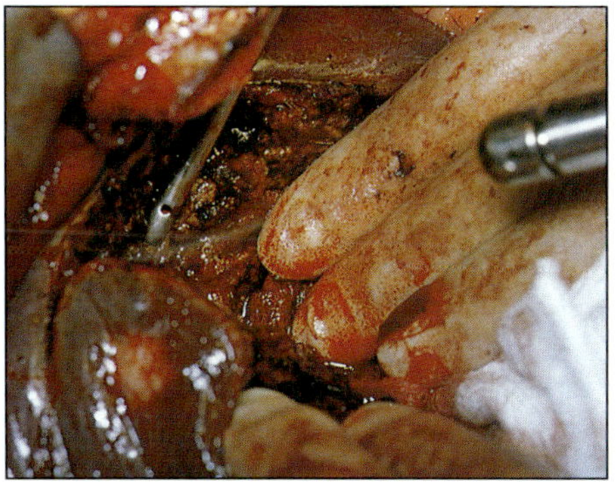 4b

4a and **b** Ultrasonic and water-jet dissectors used in hepatic resection.

Either further scanning with CT, or use of Magnetic Resonance scans enhanced with Gadolinium can be used to look for spread and multiple primaries. If none is seen, then coeliac and mesenteric angiography would be the next step both to assist in staging and to provide the surgeon with a vascular road map. In some centres a peritoneoscopy/laparoscopy would also be undertaken. In such a young patient consideration should be given to liver transplantation, although the long-term results are not as good as for parenchymal disease with a high incidence of tumour recurrence. If surgery is deemed impossible, then there are two further forms of treatment that may be offered. The first is embolisation of the tumour either alone or more usually with chemotherapy, while the second is chemotherapy alone. Unfortunately, chemotherapy has a low success rate in this form of tumour, the best drug currently being adriamycin or a close derivative. The diagnosis of a hepatocellular carcinoma can be made if there are two or more of the following. A positive biopsy, a raised alpha feto protein, a mass lesion on a scanning procedure or a positive angiogram showing tumour circulation.

This patient underwent plugged biopsy of the lesion and this confirmed the diagnosis (**5**). A plugged biopsy was used in view of the prolongation in his

5 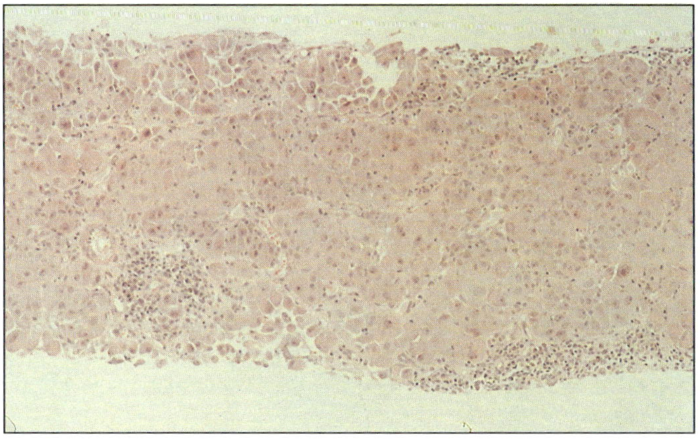

5 A biospy study.

clotting time. In this procedure a sheath is placed over the biopsy needle and after the biopsy is taken, the needle is withdrawn and gel foam is injected down the sheath as this is withdrawn from the liver (**6**).

Clinical progress

Although there was little doubt about the diagnosis in view of the massive extent of the tumour, a biopsy was undertaken. Review of the scans suggested that the tumour had invaded the diaphragm, a finding confirmed at laparotomy. Surgical resection and transplantation was thus unavailable. The patient was started on chemotherapy with adriamycin and had paracenteses performed to reduce the abdominal distension. He quite suddenly developed a large haematemesis and varices were found and injected. Review of the venous phase of his arteriogram showed tumour within the portal vein. The patient died at home after a further massive bleed.

6

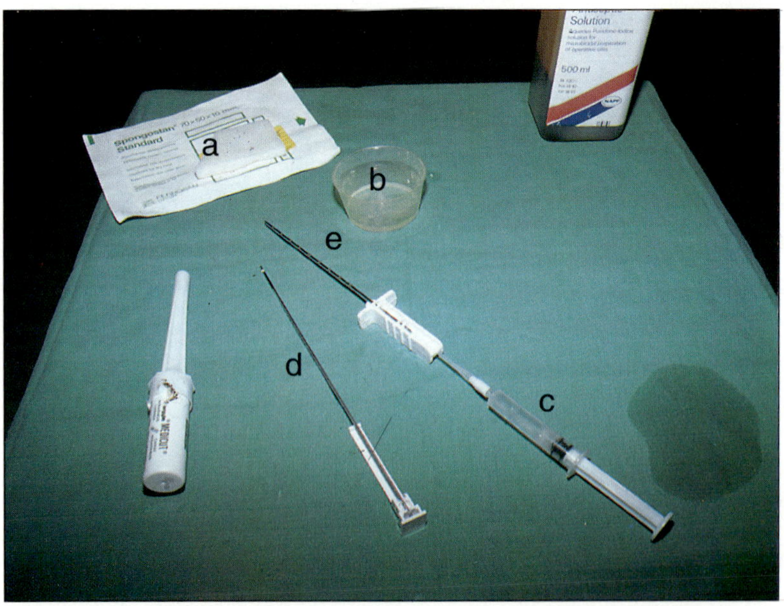

6 Plugged Biopsy Set. The fibrin foam (a) is cut into small fragments and mixed in water(b). Then it is drawn up in the syringe (c). A Trucut needle is used to take the biopsy. The inner trochar (d) is removed with the biopsy leaving the sheath (e) in place. Foam is then injected through this into the biopsy site.

Case 7

Abdominal pain and diarrhoea

This 63-year-old man presented with a history of colicky right iliac fossa pain, associated with a 3-month history of diarrhoea. There was no bleeding or weight loss. Until this time he had only suffered from asthma and this had got progressively worse in the last year. He did not smoke and drank less than 20 units of alcohol per week. He was a plethoric man who looked well and had bilateral wheezes heard throughout his chest. His abdomen was obese but despite this there was a full feeling in the right iliac fossa at the site of his pain. Rectal examination was normal.

Investigations

Haematology and Biochemistry chart on page 32; Sigmoidoscopy, see **1**; small bowel barium follow through (**2**).

1

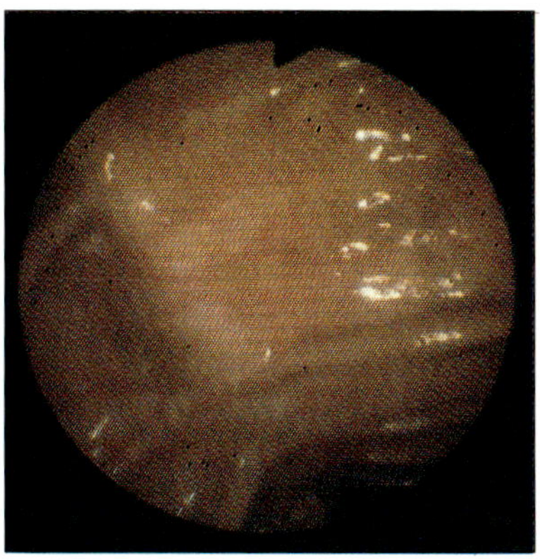

1 Sigmoidoscopy.

2

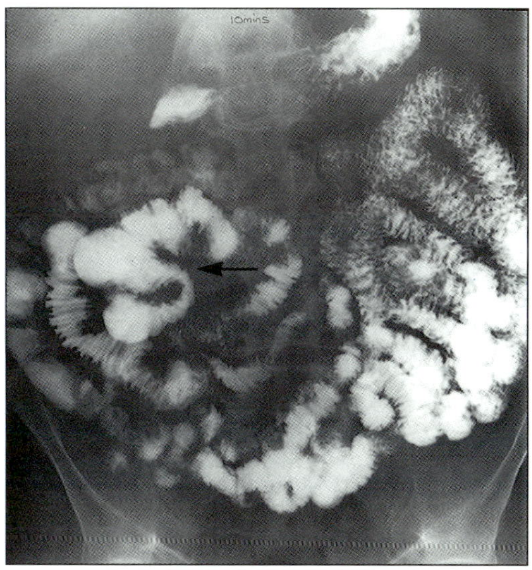

2 X-ray of the small bowel.

Questions

1 What is the differential diagnosis ?
2 Is the sigmoidoscopy normal ?
3 What does the small bowel x-ray show ?

		Normal Range			Normal Range
Hb	10.1	12.5–18 **g/dl**	**MCHC**	33.2	33–36 **g/dl**
Hct	34.1	33–47 %	**Platelets**	452	150–400/ **10^9/l**
MCV	73.1	80–100 **fl**	**WCC**	7.6	3.5–11 **/ 10^9/l**
MCH	24.4	28–33 **pg**	**ESR**	18	< 5 **mm/hr**
Sodium	138	135–145 **mmol/l**	**Blood sugar**	5.3	3.5–7.2 **mmol/l**
Potassium	3.6	3.5–5.0 **mmol/l**	**Bilirubin**	7	2–17 **mmol/l**
Chloride	101	95–105 **mmol/l**	**Alk. Phos.**	83	35–125 **U/l**
Bicarbonate	28	20–30 **mmol/l**	**ALT**	17	0–35 **U/l**
Urea	6.4	2.5–7.0 **mmol/l**	**GGT**	20	0–35 **U/l**
Creatinine	72	50–150 **mmol/l**	**Albumin**	38	36–52 **g/l**
Phosphate	1.13	0.7–1.4 **mmol/l**	**Globulin**	31	22–32 **g/l**
Calcium	2.54	2.2–2.6 **mmol/l**	**CRP**	32	5 **mg/l**

Answers and comments

1 The differential diagnosis must include a caecal or right-sided colonic carcinoma in view of the patient's symptoms, low haemoglobin, microcytosis and raised CRP level. In addition, terminal ileal disease would give the same symptoms, signs and investigation results. The commonest terminal ileal disease in the developed world would be either Crohn's disease or tuberculosis, depending upon the country and ethnic origin of the patient. This patient was a caucasian. Other forms of terminal ileal disease are much less common, such as actinomycosis or a terminal ileal tumour. A retrocaecal appendix abscess can mimic a tumour in this area.

2 The sigmoidoscopy was entirely normal and a good view was obtained of the normal fine vasculature.

3 A double contrast barium enema showed no significant abnormality; however the small bowel x-ray (**2**) shows an irregular narrowed segment of terminal ileum (arrow) with possible ulceration and some proximal dilatation. There was the suggestion of an adjacent skip lesion. The radiologist reported this as consistent with terminal ileal Crohn's disease.

Further clinical details

The patient was started on a short course of steroids for the presumed Crohn's disease and noted an improvement in his pain. The diarrhoea did not alter. After 4 weeks treatment the patient developed a severe attack of asthma and requested his general practitioner to make a home visit. Apart from the asthma the patient was noted to have a florid dusky purple colouration of his face, hands and chest wall.

Questions

4 What should you ask the patient?
5 What further investigations would be indicated ?
6 What other features of the syndrome would you look for?
7 What are the other causes of this syndrome ?

Answers and comments

4 In view of the skin colouration, the patient should be asked if he had experienced any attacks of flushing and whether these were associated with any exacerbation of his asthma. In fact for about 2 months he had noted bouts of flushing lasting from 4 seconds to several minutes. He thought the attacks were increasing in frequency and noted that during the severe flushes his chest got tighter. Figure **3** shows the typical flush which can be transient or fixed.
5 The investigation required to make the diagnosis of carcinoid syndrome is a 24-hour urine for 5 HIAA (5 Hydroxy–Indole–Acetic–Acid). This is the breakdown product of 5 Hydroxy–Tryptamine. This patient's result was 1500 mg/24 hours, with an upper limit of normal of 60 mg/24 hours.
6 The other clinical feature is a pulmonary stenotic murmur, which this patient did not have.
7 Although a small-bowel tumour is the commonest site, carcinoid tumours can occur anywhere in the GI tract. They are commonly found in the appendix and less commonly in the colon and stomach.The syndrome is only seen if there are either secondary deposits in the liver from a malignant gastrointestinal carcinoid, or if a carcinoid tumour drains its venous supply directly into the systemic circulation, such as can occur with bronchial or gonadal tumours. In view of the biochemical results a CT scan was performed of this patient's liver (**4**).

3

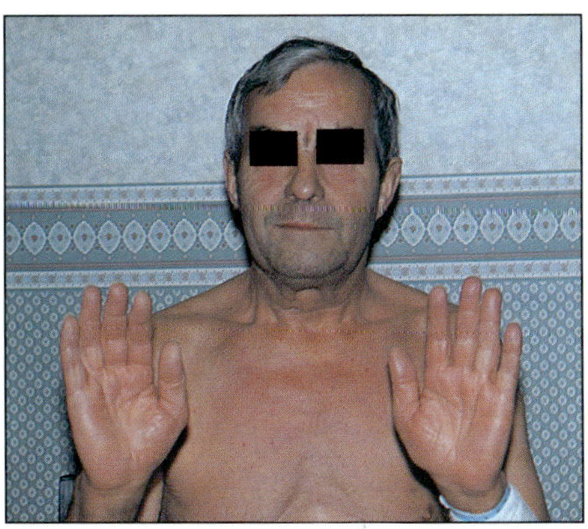

3 Note patient's skin colour.

4

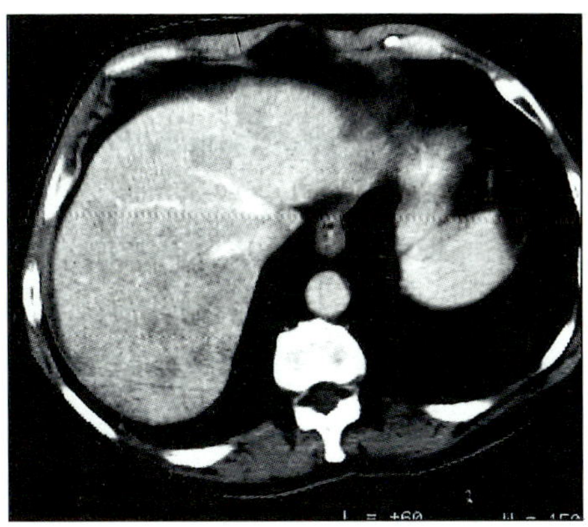

4 CT liver scan.

Questions

8 What does the CT scan show?
9 What treatment would you use on this patient ?

Answers and comments

8 The CT scan shows multiple lucent areas throughout the liver with gross replacement of the left lobe by tumour tissue. On review of his abdominal findings the liver edge was just palpable below the costal margin.

9 Surgical resection of the primary tumour would only be indicated if it were causing obstructive symptoms. Surgery would not be easy as this type of active tumour induces an intense desmoplastic reaction, which almost certainly caused some of the appearances seen on the small bowel x-ray. In the presence of so many secondary deposits surgical cure was not possible. Initial therapy is aimed at blocking the effects of 5HT and other vasoactive substances secreted by these tumours. Drugs such as cyproheptidine may help with the diarrhoea as does methysergide, but recently the use of long-acting somatostatin analogues such as octreotide has dramatically improved symptom control. The drug has to be given 2 or 3 times a day and the injection site can hurt. In this patient his symptoms dramatically settled with no further diarrhoea and complete suppression of his flushing. His asthma remained the same with no further deterioration.

Clinical progress

Over the next year his symptoms were controlled by gradually increasing doses of octreotide such that by the end of that time he required 500 mcg injections to control them. Gradually his symptoms escaped control with frequent watery stools as well as marked facial flushing. At this stage it was decided to try and reduce the tumour bulk by embolising some of the liver metastases. By superselective arteriography one of three branches of his hepatic artery was embolised using metal coils (**5**). This was performed after careful preparation of the patient to avoid a carcinoid crisis and with antibiotics to prevent the infarcted tissues from becoming infected. This produced dramatic improvement in his symptoms and he was able to get off the octreotide completely for several months with no symptoms at all. Gradually the flushing has returned and he has restarted the octreotide at a dose of 50 mcg b.d. Further embolisation will take place if management again becomes difficult.

5

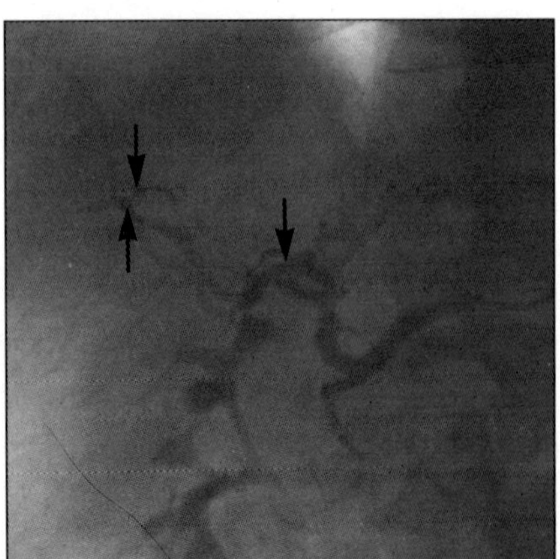

5 Embolisation of branches of the right hepatic artery with metal coils (arrows).

Case 8

Elderly man with recurrent anaemia and melaena

This pleasant, fit 76-year-old was referred from a small hospital with the history that he had become anaemic on several occasions. His haemoglobin had dropped to 7.6 g/dl on one occasion and he had multiple blood transfusions, with a total of 32 units being transfused over 3 years. He had had several investigations in the past. Three separate upper gastrointestinal endoscopies had been performed and he was said to have gastritis. A barium enema was performed, which is shown in **1**. A flexible sigmoidoscopy to the splenic flexure did not reveal anything diagnostically. Apart from prostatism he was well. On the last admission he had passed several black, tarry stools. On examination he was a fit, overweight man with an abnormal tongue and lips (**2**) and abnormal nails (**3**).

Investigations

Haematology and Biochemistry chart on page 36; Barium enema, see **1.**

Questions

1 What are the lesions on his lips and tongue?
2 What further questions would you ask to fully elucidate the history?
3 What is the significance of his nails?
4 What further investigations would you undertake?
5 What forms of treatment are available?

1

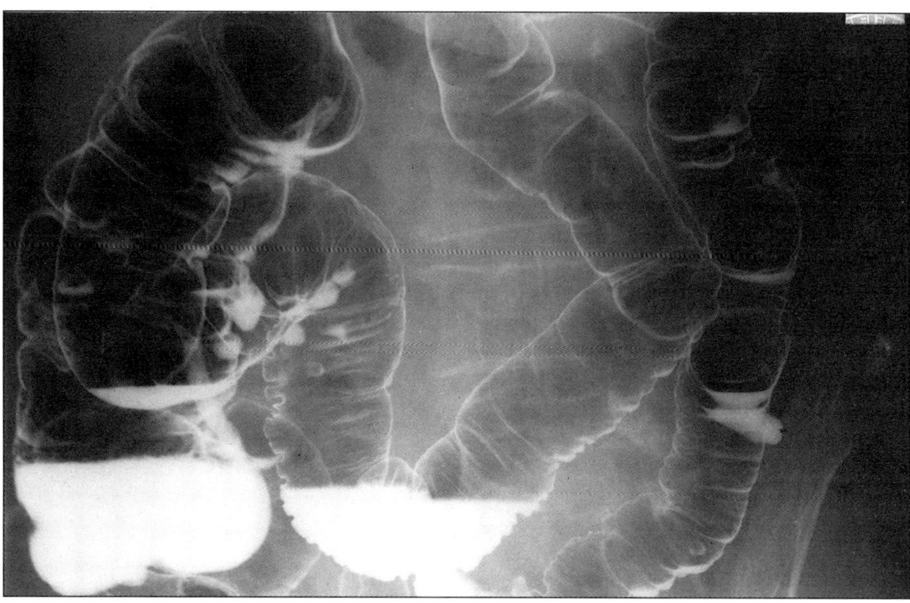

1 Barium enema shows only divertivular disease.

2 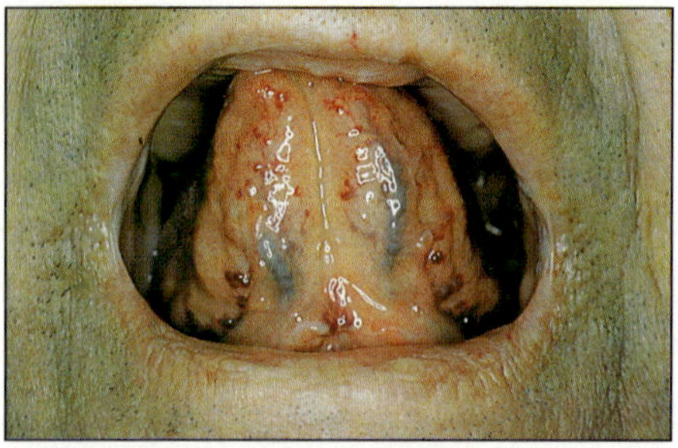

2 Abnormal tongue and lips.

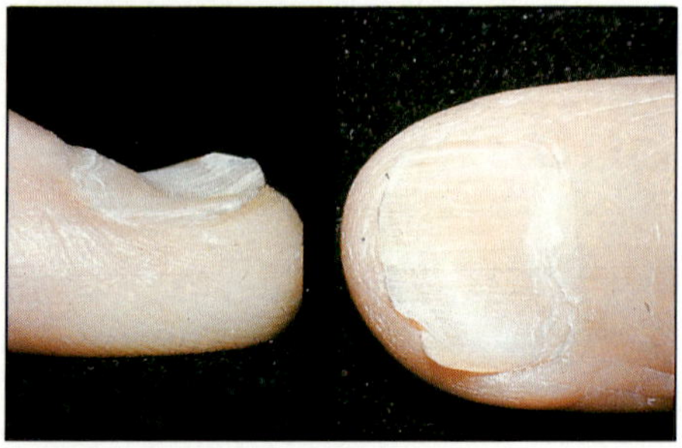 3

3 Abnormal nails.

		Normal Range			Normal Range
Hb	9.7	12.5–18 **g/dl**	**MCHC**	34.3	33–36 **g/dl**
Hct	29.1	33–47 %	**Platelets**	264	150–400/ **10^9/l**
MCV	73.6	80–100 **fl**	**WCC**	6.1	3.5–11 **/ 10^9/l**
MCH	26.1	28–33 **pg**	**ESR**	9	< 5 **mm/hr**
Sodium	142	135–145 **mmol/l**	**Blood sugar**	3.8	3.5–7.2 **mmol/l**
Potassium	4.0	3.5–5.0 **mmol/l**	**Bilirubin**	8	2–17 **mmol/l**
Chloride	109	95–105 **mmol/l**	**Alk. Phos.**	86	35–125 **U/l**
Bicarbonate	24	20–30 **mmol/l**	**ALT**	25	0–35 **U/l**
Urea	4.1	2.5–7.0 **mmol/l**	**GGT**	30	0–35 **U/l**
Creatinine	52	50–150 **mmol/l**	**Albumin**	45	36–52 **g/l**
Phosphate	1.05	0.7–1.4 **mmol/l**	**Globulin**	28	22–32 **g/l**
Calcium	2.43	2.2–2.6 **mmol/l**	**CRP**	<5	< 5 **mg/l**

Answers and comments

1 The lesions shown are telangiectatic spots.
2 It is important to ask if the patient had a history of epistaxis, haemoptysis or haematuria. For many years he had suffered from recurrent epistaxes but there was no other history of bleeding, with the exception of the single episode of melaena. A careful family history revealed that his mother, one sister and one of his daughters had similar lesions on their lips, and several members of the family had had recurrent nose bleeds. It thus appeared that this patient had hereditary haemorrhagic telangiectasia otherwise known as Osler–Rendu–Weber Syndrome.
3 He has koilonychia due to iron deficiency, presumably caused by recurrent episodes of occult bleeding. Occasionally koilonychia can be seen confined to one or two nails, and when this is seen it is probably the result of repetitive pressure on that nail as part of an occupation.
4 It is clearly important to assess the extent of the telangiectasia to determine if this is localised to one area within the GI tract or whether it is more gene-

ralised. The first step would be to repeat the upper gastrointestinal endoscopy, because frequently telangiectasia is misinterpreted as gastritis by inexperienced endoscopists. If this was clear, then a small-bowel enteroscopy would be the next investigation. There are several types of small-bowel enteroscopes now available. One type is the Sonde type (**4**) which is a non-steerable transnasal floppy scope which passes through the GI tract by using an inflatable balloon to stimulate peristalsis. Although this can traverse the entire small bowel, the procedure is time-consuming, the view on extubation is limited and it is not possible to undertake therapy through it. The other main type is the Push enteroscope which is an elongated, floppy gastroscope (**5**) which can be steered, and through which therapy can be delivered. This scope generally only reaches the mid jejunum but can on occasion get into the ileum. Whenever there is thought to be bleeding from the lower bowel, a full colonoscopy is much better at finding the cause of bleeding than a barium enema and sigmoidoscopy. This is particularly the case when vascular lesions such as telangiectasia or angiodysplasia are sought. This patient underwent full colonoscopy 2 days after his small-bowel enteroscopy and the result is shown in **6**. Figure **7** shows a small-bowel endoscopy of a telangiectatic spot. If the patient presents with a massive gastrointestinal bleed and endoscopy is not possible because of the volume of blood seen, then mesenteric angiography may show an area of angiodysplasia and/or identify the bleeding site.

4

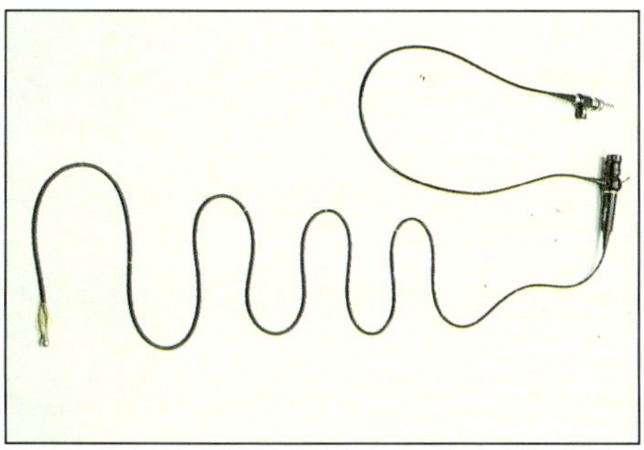

4 Sonde type enteroscope.

5

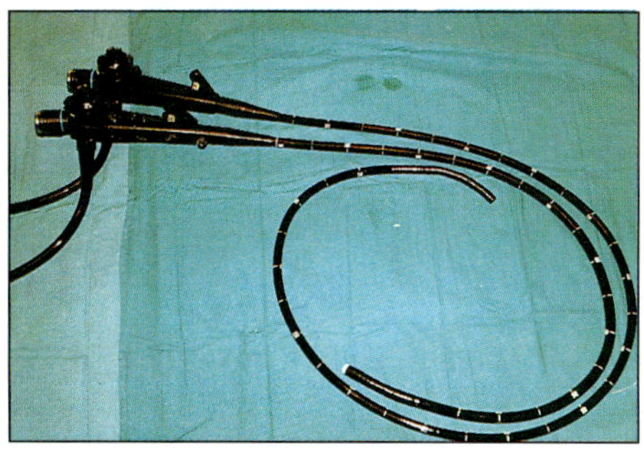

5 Push type enteroscope.

6

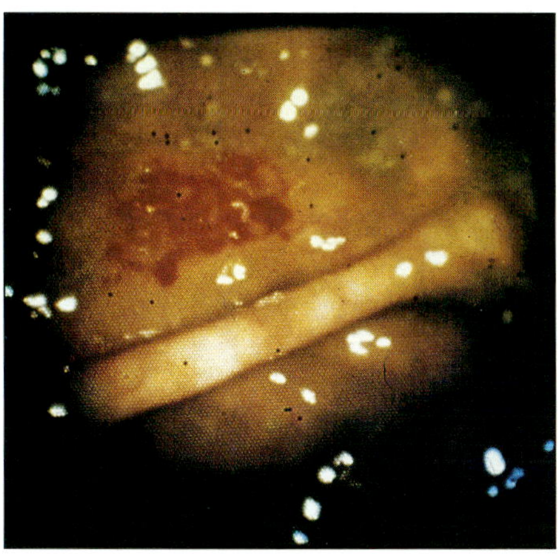

6 Result of colonoscopy.

7

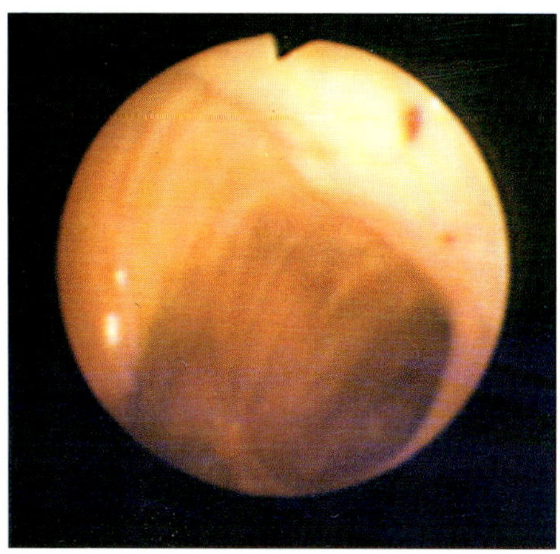

7 Endoscopic view of the small bowel.

5 The treatment offered to the patient depends upon the severity of the bleeding, the anatomical extent of the lesions, the facilities that are available and the patient's overall fitness. For massive bleeding, angiography followed by surgery and removal of the site of bleeding may be the only way to stop the haemorrhage. For smaller bleeds or occult bleeding presenting as anaemia, then the extent of the vascular lesion should be determined. The possibilities for treatment would be endoscopic ablation (with laser, diathermy or sclerotherapy), localised resection, or in the case of difficult lesions, hormone therapy. Generally, for localised lesions in the stomach, small bowel or colon, endoscopic therapy should be attempted first. If after a reasonable trial of endoscopic therapy bleeding persists, then surgery should be considered if the patient is fit enough. For those patients with extensive lesions affecting more than one anatomical site, or for those patients who are not fit for surgery, a significant benefit has been shown by the administration of oestrogen and progesterone in the form of norethisterone and ethinyloestradiol.

Clinical progress

Small telangiectatic lesions were seen in the upper small bowel, but large bleeding lesions were visualised in the caecum. These were initially hot biopsied and have subsequently been treated by laser therapy.The advantage of laser treatment for such lesions is that the laser is applied at a distance from the lesion (a few millimetres) and thus the laser fibre is not in contact with the vascular abnormality. With all other endoscopically delivered therapy the probe is in contact with the lesion and any coagulum formed can be pulled off as the probe is removed, or bleeding can be induced simply by touching the lesion.

Case 9

Weak legs and oedema

This 53-year-old patient was referred by his general practitioner with the history that he had noticed his legs were getting numb and he kept tripping over objects. He noticed that his ankles had also been getting swollen for a few weeks and that he was experiencing excessive thirst and had polyuria and nocturia and frequency. He drank 32 units of alcohol per week but did not smoke. His father had died in his 50s from liver disease, and had been a heavy drinker. The patient lived alone and had no other family except an elderly mother. On examination he was generally pigmented (**1**) with 8 cm hepatomegaly and a palpable spleen. There was a trace of ankle oedema and he had a ' stocking' distribution sensory loss to mid-calf bilaterally with some degree of bilateral foot-drop. Bedside urine testing showed ++++ sugar.

Investigations

Haematology and Biochemistry charts on page 40. Radiology: CT scan of liver(**2**); Liver biopsy: (**3** and **4**).

Questions

1 What is the abnormality shown on the CT scan?
2 What does the liver biopsy show and what stain is used ?
3 What confirmatory blood tests should be undertaken ?
4 What management is required for this patient ?

1

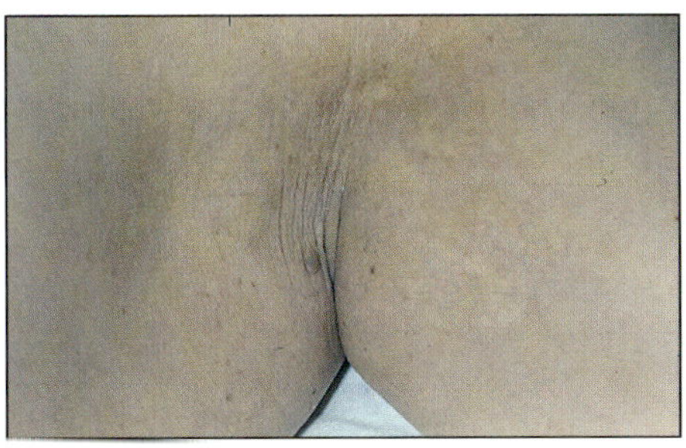

1 Patient's axilla showing pigmentation and hair loss.

2

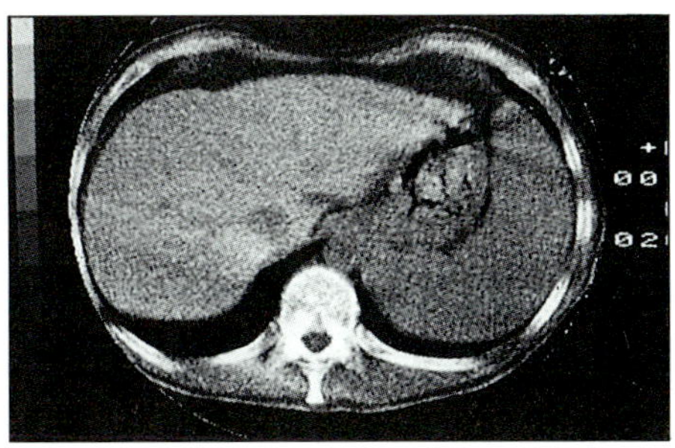

2 CT scan of the liver.

3

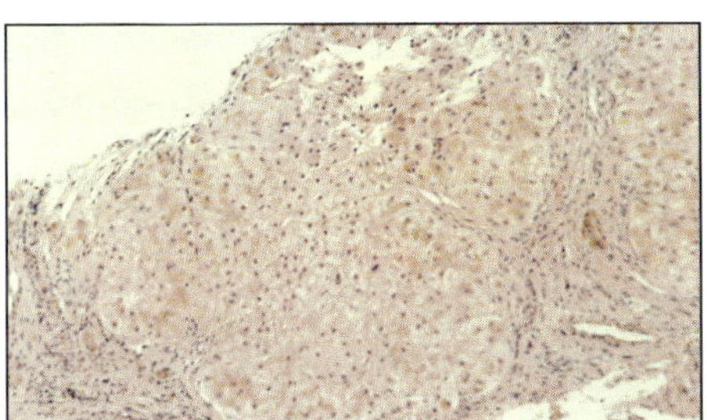

4

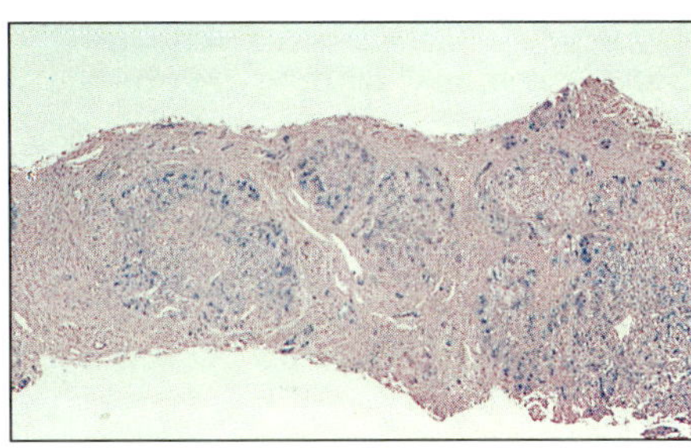

3 and **4** Studies of two separate biopsies.

		Normal Range			Normal Range
Hb	14.2	12.5–18 **g/dl**	**MCHC**	34.0	33–36 **g/dl**
Hct	42.6	33–47 **%**	**Platelets**	202	150–400/ **10^9/l**
MCV	87.7	80–100 **fl**	**WCC**	6.4	3.5–11 **/ 10^9/l**
MCH	29.9	28–33 **pg**	**ESR**	3	< 20 **mm/hr**
Sodium	140	135–145 **mmol/l**	**Blood sugar**	24.6	3.5–7.2 **mmol/l**
Potassium	3.5	3.5–5.0 **mmol/l**	**Bilirubin**	63	2–17 **mmol/l**
Chloride	98	95–105 **mmol/l**	**Alk. Phos.**	324	35–125 **U/l**
Bicarbonate	26	20–30 **mmol/l**	**ALT**	120	0–35 **U/l**
Urea	2.6	2.5–7.0 **mmol/l**	**GGT**	159	0–35 **U/l**
Creatinine	73	50–150 **mmol/l**	**Albumin**	28	36–52 **g/l**
Phosphate	1.35	0.7–1.4 **mmol/l**	**Globulin**	34	22–32 **g/l**
Calcium	2.24	2.2–2.6 **mmol/l**	**CRP**	6	< 5 **mg/l**

Answers and comments

1 The CT liver scan shows that the liver is of higher density than the other soft tissues. This is an unenhanced scan and signifies heavy iron overload in the liver, which renders it denser to x-rays. The scan also shows a grossy enlarged spleen. In **5**, **6** and **7** a normal liver is compared with that of a haemochromatotic liver and a liver with gross fatty changes.

2 The haematoxylin and eosin stain shows disorganised liver structure with nodules and fibrosis. There is also a brown pigment seen predominately in the hepatocytes. The special stain is a Perle's stain for iron showing marked iron deposition. Apart from haemachromatosis the only other condition that might produce a similar picture is iron overload in an alcoholic, or transfusion siderosis. There was no history of recurrent transfusions but the patient did consume an excessive amount of alcohol. The lack of fat on the liver biopsy and the extent of the iron deposition favoured the cause being haemochromatosis. A biopsy from an alcoholic with iron overload is shown in **8** for comparison.

3 The patient had his serum iron, iron binding capacity and % saturation measured as well as his serum ferritin. The results are shown in the table on page 41.

5

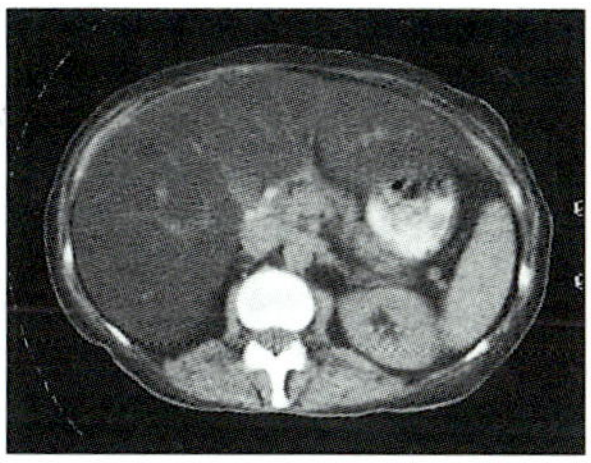

5 Fatty liver.

6

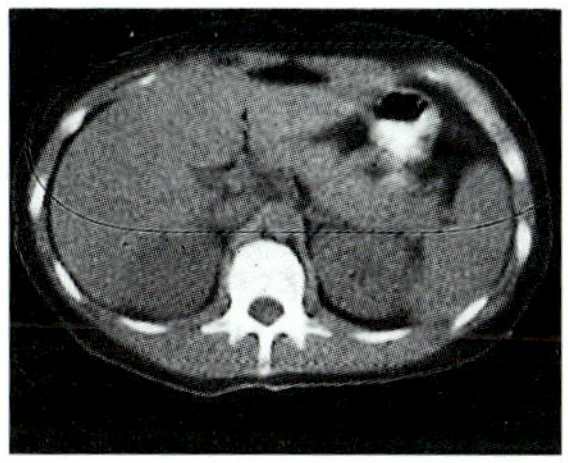

6 Normal liver.

7

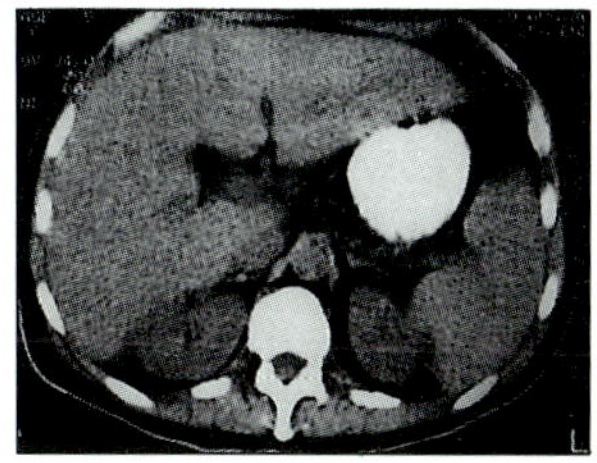

7 Haemochromatosis.

Note that the normal liver has the same density as spleen and kidneys.

8

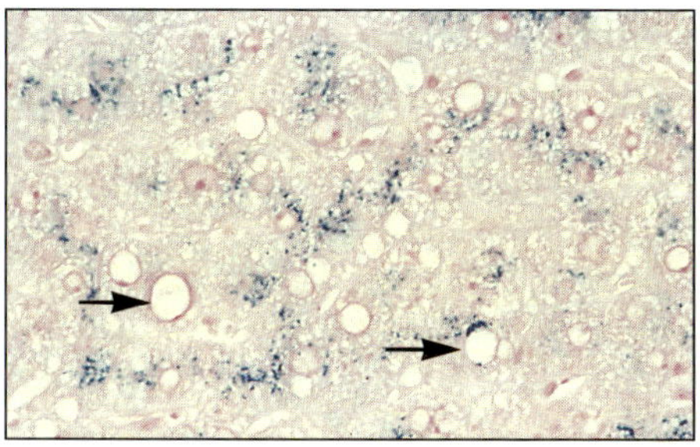

8 Alcoholic live disease showing fatty infiltration (arrows).

		Normal
Serum Fe	2.3	13.32 **μmol/l**
TIBC	174	64–106 **μmol/l**
Ferritin	10	19–300 **Mg/l**
ARTERIAL BLOOD GASES		
pH	7.41	7.38–7.44**KPa**
pCO_2	4.8	4.7–6.00**KPa**
pO_2	11.5	1.3–14.0 **KPa**
Standard bicarb	23	22–26 **μmol/l**
Base excess	–1	–2.3–+2.3 **μmol/l**

These showed the patient to be fully saturated with a very high ferritin level. If difficulty still occurs in trying to differentiate between an alcoholic with overload and a true haemochromatotic, then measurement of liver iron is the investigation of choice.

4 Management involves treatment of his diabetes, definition of the type and extent of the liver disease and removal of iron. In addition, if there were any siblings or children, they should be screened for evidence of iron overload.

Clinical progress

The patient's diabetes was quickly and rapidly controlled by twice daily insulin. On this regimen his peripheral neuropathy completely resolved. Iron was removed by weekly venesection until he had become mildly anaemic with iron deficiency. He has been advised to avoid foods with high iron content. Regular checks of his iron, ferritin and alpha fetoprotein are made. In some units a repeat liver biopsy is undertaken to confirm desaturation.

Case 10

Dyspepsia and diarrhoea

This 48-year-old farm auctioneer presented with a 3-month history of indigestion and heartburn as well as a 5-month history of diarrhoea and 7 kg weight loss. He was opening his bowels up to 6 times a day and had occasionally noticed undigested food. There was no blood in the stools and he had no abdominal pain. He complained of occasional night sweats. Six years earlier he had developed renal colic and had passed several stones. During investigation of these he was found to be hypercalcaemic and had a parathyroid adenoma removed. He had no further urinary symptoms and repeat checks on his calcium levels had been normal. On examination he was fit and had no abnormal signs except for his parathyroidectomy scar.

Investigations

Haematology and Biochemistry chart on page 43. Endoscopy: Lower oesophagus (**1**); Duodenum (**2**); The small bowel x-ray showed general dilation of the bowel without fold thickening and with some dilution of the barium. The appearances where said to be non-specific and consistent with malabsorption.

1

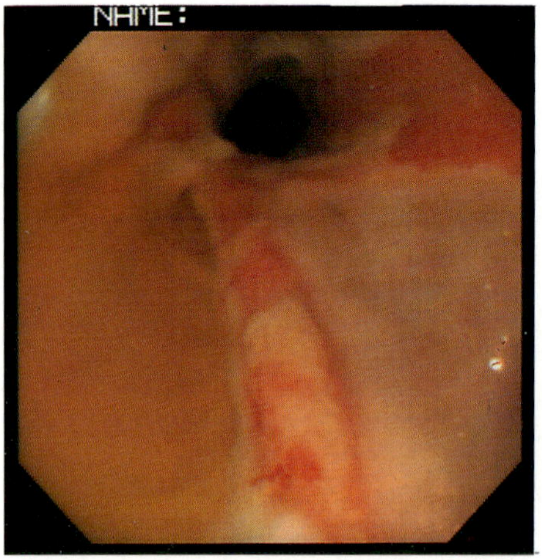

1 Endoscopy: lower oesophagus

2

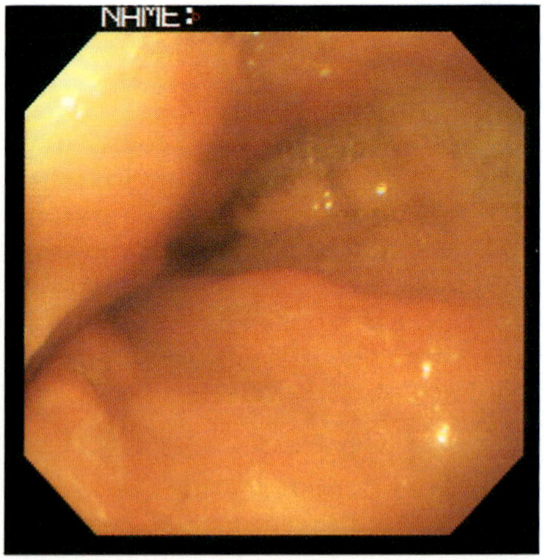

2 Endoscopy: duodenum.

Questions

1 What do the endoscopies show?
2 What conditions need to be excluded in view of his work ?
3 What are the possible causes of his diarrhoea ?
4 How would you further investigate him ?

		Normal Range			Normal Range
Hb	14.6	12.5–18.0 **g/dl**	**MCHC**	34.4	33–36 **g/dl**
Hct	42.3	33–47 **%**	**Platelets**	153	150–400/ **10^9/l**
MCV	87.8	80–100 **fl**	**WCC**	7.8	3.5–11 **/ 10^9/l**
MCH	30.3	28–33 **pg**	**ESR**	8	< 10 **mm/hr**
Sodium	143	135–145 **mmol/l**	**Blood sugar**	4.2	3.5–7.2 **mmol/l**
Potassium	4.0	3.5–5.0 **mmol/l**	**Bilirubin**	4	2–17 **mmol/l**
Chloride	105	95–105 **mmol/l**	**Alk. Phos.**	82	35–125 **U/l**
Bicarbonate	26	20–30 **mmol/l**	**ALT**	23	0–35 **U/l**
Urea	5.3	2.5–7.0 **mmol/l**	**GGT**	17	0–35 **U/l**
Creatinine	95	50–150 **mmol/l**	**Albumin**	43	36–52 **g/l**
Phosphate	1.08	0.7–1.4 **mmol/l**	**Globulin**	22	22–32 **g/l**
Calcium	2.29	2.2–2.6 **mmol/l**	**CRP**	<5	5 **mg/l**

Answers and comments

1 The lower end of the oesophagus shows inflammation and discrete ulceration (Grade 2 Oesophagitis) consistent with reflux oesophagitis. The duodenum was inflamed and contained several apthoid ulcers or erosions.
The stomach, apart from containing a lot of resting gastric juice, looked normal.
2 In view of his work with farm animals and the history of night sweats Tuberculosis, Brucellosis, and Q fever all needed to be excluded. All tests for these and other infectious diseases were negative.
3 We are thus left with a patient with oesophagitis and duodenitis with unexplained weight loss and diarrhoea. The small bowel x-ray did not show any features of Crohn's disease nor any focal abnormality to suggest a localised lymphoma or tuberculosis. However, other small-bowel pathology needs to be excluded including coeliac disease, small-bowel lymphoma and Whipple's disease. The presence of both oesophagitis and duodenitis, together with the large volume of resting gastric juice, in a patient with a history of previous parathyroid adenoma , should suggest that a hypersecretory state may be present such as the Zollinger–Ellison syndrome. In view of the weight loss and diarrhoea, colonic disease also needs exculsion.
4 At the time of his endoscopy biopsies of the small bowel were taken that were entirely normal. A colonoscopy was undertaken which was similarly normal. A fasting plasma gastrin and GI Hormone profile was requested and the results were as follows: Vasoactive intestinal polypeptide (VIP) 11 (N < 30 pmol/l); Pancreatic polypeptide (PP) 206 (N < 300 pmol/l); Gastrin 96 (N < 40 pmol/l); Glucagon 81 (N < 50 pmol/l); Neurotensin 36 (N < 100 pmol/l).

Questions

5 What are the causes of hypergastrinaemia ?
6 How would you investigate this patient further?

Answers and comments

5 There are many causes of hypergastrinaemia, although most do not apply to this patient. Thus pernicious anaemia causes gross elevation of gastrin due to the anacidity in the stomach. This patient had gastric acid present and in addition had evidence of peptic damage at least in part due to acid. The patient was not on any acid lowering drug , nor had there been any previous gastric surgery or small bowel resection. His renal function was normal and there was no other obvious cause for the hypergastrinaemia.

6 Investigation should be aimed at confirming the presence of hypergastrinaemia and trying to find the underlying cause. The confirmation of the Zollinger–Ellison (ZE) syndrome is made by initially confirming the presence of increased gastric acid secretion, and then in this case where gastrin levels were not grossly elevated using stimulation tests of gastrin secretion. Once the diagnosis is confirmed, then a detailed investigation of the pancreas and duodenum should be made to look for evidence of either single or multiple tumours and any evidence of metastases. Up to 60% of ZE tumours are malignant. In view of this patient's history The Multiple Endocrine Neoplasia Syndrome Type I is a possibility and investigation of his pituitary would be sensible. Family screening should also be considered.

Investigations

Secretin stimulation test (**3**); Gastric acid secretion studies (**4**).

Questions

7 What does the acid output study demonstrate ?
8 What does the secretin study suggest?
9 What further investigation is indicated and how would you treat this patient?

3

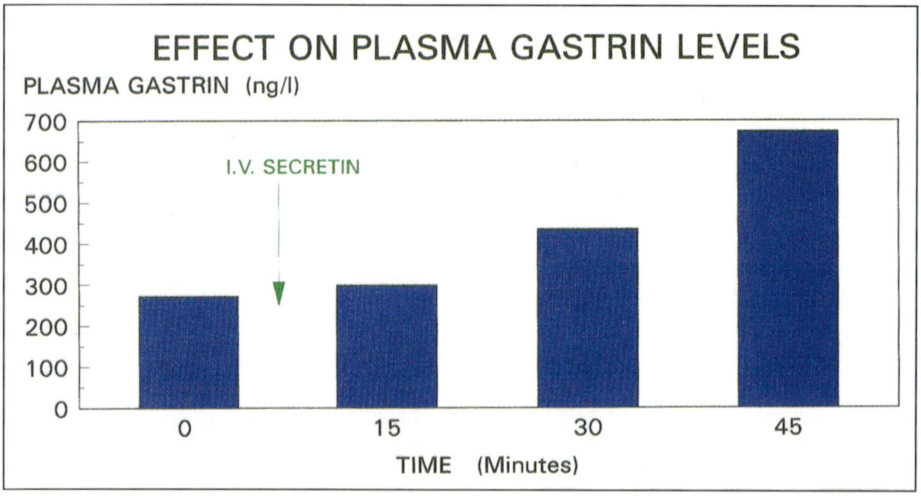

3 Secreting stimulation test.

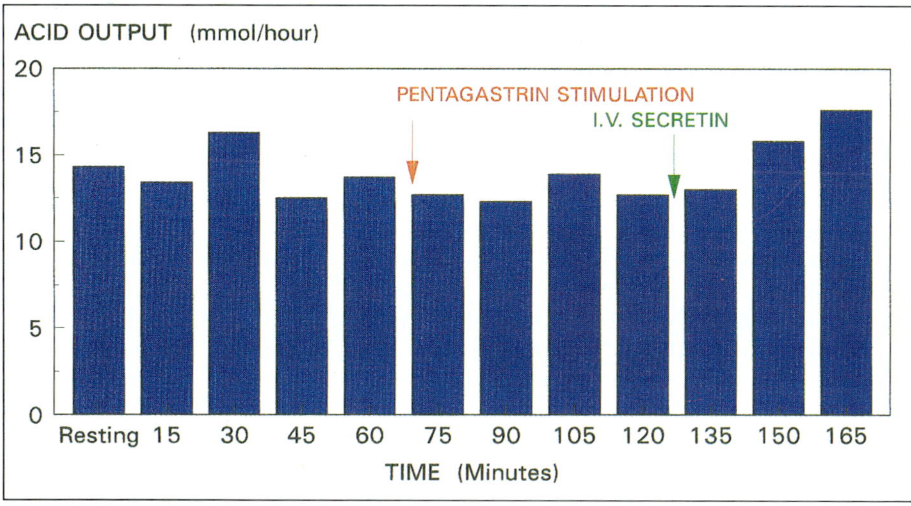

4

4 Gastric acid secretion studies.

Answers and comments

7 The acid output study on this patient shows high basal acid secretion of 52.4 mmol/hour (upper limit of normal 6 mmol/hour). Basal secretion is calculated as twice the lowest 30 minute output. The maximal acid output in this patient was 53.2 mmol/hour (upper limit of normal 40 mmol/hour) and this is calculated as twice the peak half hour output.This patient thus has a stomach that is producing a large amount of acid under basal conditions, which when stimulated by Pentagastrin does not produce a further rise in output as would happen in an unstimulated stomach. The ratio of Basal Acid Output to Maximal Acid Output (BAO/MAO) was 0.98. A value of greater than 0.6 is suggestive of a gastrinoma.The administration of intravenous secretin produced a slight increase in acid output which is again a finding in patients with a gastrinoma.

8 The secretin study demonstrates a more than doubling of the gastrin level in response to a bolus of intravenous secretin, although the response was a little delayed. A 100% increase in plasma gastrin within 30 minutes of the injection is said to be a positive test, indicating a gastrinoma. The secretin test is a quicker and easier test than the calcium infusion test which is also used in some centres.These tests are used when the basal fasting plasma gastrin is not greatly elevated. Values over 300 ng/l are usually diagnostic in the absence of achlorhydria.

9 Having thus established the diagnosis as being that of the Zollinger–Ellison syndrome in a patient with Multiple Endocrine Neoplasia Type I, the next aim of investigation is to look for the adenoma or tumour. A contrast enhanced CT scan would probably be the next step followed by coeliac and mesenteric angiography. If no identifiable lesion is seen, then transhepatic portal venous sampling can be used to look for the site of gastrin secretion. Endoscopic ultrasound is said by some to be the best method to look for small adenomas in the pancreas.

Clinical progress

This patient underwent both CT scanning and visceral angiography and it was not possible to see a lesion. Rather than subject him to a blind pancreatic resection, it is planned that he will have repeated investigations performed regularly. In the past the only way to protect the patient from the excess gastric secretion was for the patient either to have a pancreatectomy or a total gastrectomy. Both operations carry a significant mortality and morbidity. The advent of Histamine H_2 Receptor Blockade enabled many patients to be rendered asymptomatic while either awaiting surgery or when surgery was not indicated, as for instance when no lesion could be found or when there is evidence of multiple metastases. More recently the introduction of Proton Pump Inhibitors has further revolutionised these patients' management by switching off acid secretion. This patient has been rendered totally asymptomatic by omeprazole 40 mg daily.The diarrhoea so often seen in the Z–E syndrome is due to the high level of acid secretion damaging the intestinal mucosa as well as inactivation of pancreatic enzymes within the small-bowel lumen giving rise to malabsorption. A recently developed new technique is to scan the patient after the administration of Indium labelled Octreotide (a somatostatin analogue) (**5**), which highlights hormone producing tumours in the pancreas.

5

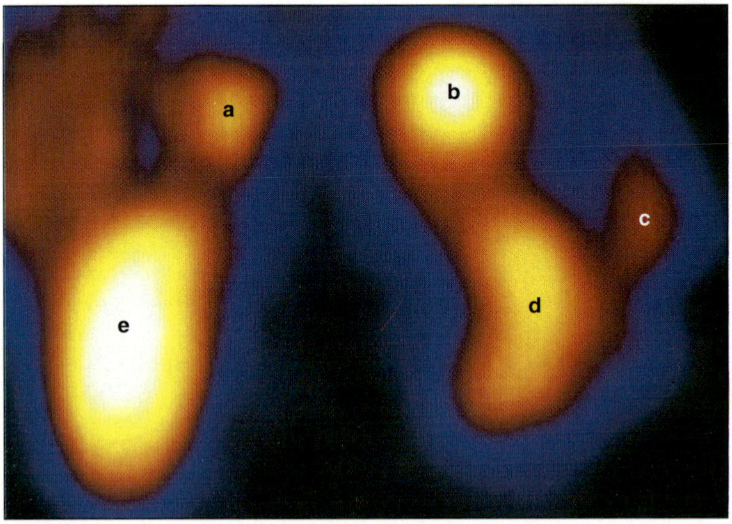

5 Indium labelled octreotide scan: a = liver, b = tumour, c = spleen, d = left kidney, e = right kidney.

Case 11

Ulcer on leg and diarrhoea

After a long history of diarrhoea, this unemployed male aged 56, visited the local homeopathic clinic complaining not only of his diarrhoea but also of an enlarging ulcerated area on his leg (**1**). He was admitted to the homeopathic ward but despite regular dressings and homeopathic treatment his condition deteriorated. He informed the staff that he had been diagnosed as having colitis some 20 years previously but had never been fully investigated or followed up. During his admission his diarrhoea increased and he noticed blood mixed with the stool for the first time. He was started on prednisolone 5 mg per day but showed no improvement; he was referred to the Gastroenterology Unit for advice. On examination his abdomen was soft and non-tender but there was a full feeling in the left iliac fossa.

Investigations

Haematology and Biochemistry chart on page 48. Plain x-ray of abdomen (**2**).

1

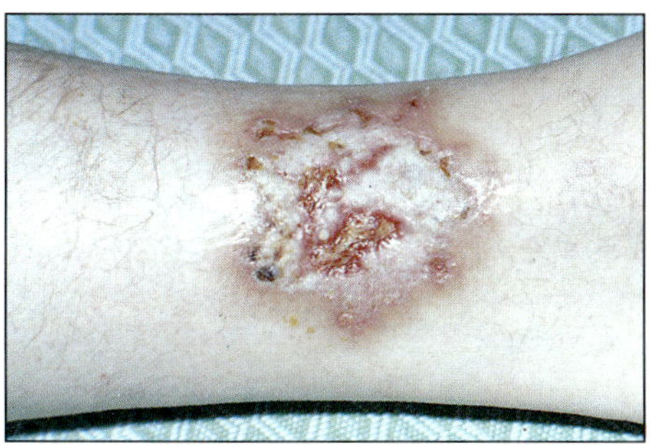

1 Ulceration of the leg.

2

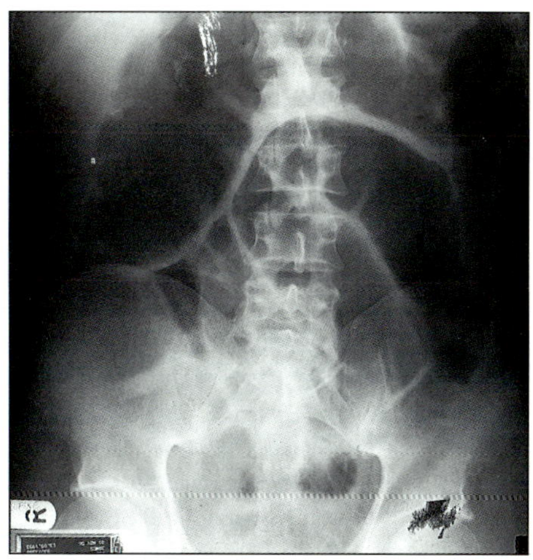

2 Plain x-ray of the abdomen.

Questions

1 What is the skin lesion ?
2 What other skin lesions can be associated with colitis ?
3 What does the plain x-ray show?
4 What are the best indicators of disease severity ?

Case 11

		Normal Range			Normal Range
Hb	7.3	12.5–18 **g/dl**	**MCHC**	29.3	33–36 **g/dl**
Hct	24.1	33–47 %	**Platelets**	556	150–400/ **10^9/l**
MCV	55.1	80–100 **fl**	**WCC**	9.0	3.5–11 **/ 10^9/l**
MCH	16.1	28–33 **pg**	**ESR**	56	< 20 **mm/hr**
Sodium	141	135–145 **mmol/l**	**Blood sugar**	3.3	3.5–7.2 **mmol/l**
Potassium	3.8	3.5–5.0 **mmol/l**	**Bilirubin**	8	2–17 **mmol/l**
Chloride	98	95–105 **mmol/l**	**Alk. Phos.**	86	35–125 **U/l**
Bicarbonate	22	20–30 **mmol/l**	**ALT**	17	0–35 **U/l**
Urea	6.1	2.5–7.0 **mmol/l**	**GGT**	16	0–35 **U/l**
Creatinine	119	50–150 **mmol/l**	**Albumin**	25	36–52 **g/l**
Phosphate	0.98	0.7–1.4 **mmol/l**	**Globulin**	36	22–32 **g/l**
Calcium	2.49	2.2–2.6 **mmol/l**	**CRP**	5	<5 **mg/l**

Answers and comments

1 The lesion is pyoderma gangrenosum. This can occur without the presence of inflammatory bowel disease but in more than 50% of cases is associated with either ulcerative colitis or Crohn's disease.

2 More common than pyoderma gangrenosum is erythema nodosum. Again this is not specific to ulcerative colitis (**3**). A vasculitic rash is sometimes seen in association with inflammatory bowel disease. However, the occurrence of such a rash in a patient with bloody diarrhoea should raise the question of Henoch–Schonlein Purpura .

3 The plain x-ray shows large bowel distension with islands of mucosal oedema. The appearances are of total colitis, but measurement of colonic width did not suggest toxin dilatation (more than 8 cm in the transverse colon).

4 The important clinical features that suggest severe disease are pulse rate, temperature, stool frequency, white-cell count and serum albumin. In addition the degree of anaemia suggests that there has been considerable bleeding from the bowel in the absence of any other cause.This patient was apyrexial but had a moderate tachycardia and on admission was emptying his bowels more than 10 times in 24 hours. The low-serum albumin also signified that this was a severe attack.

Questions

5 What further investigation is important ?
6 How would you treat this patient?
7 What are the indications for surgery in ulcerative colitis?

3

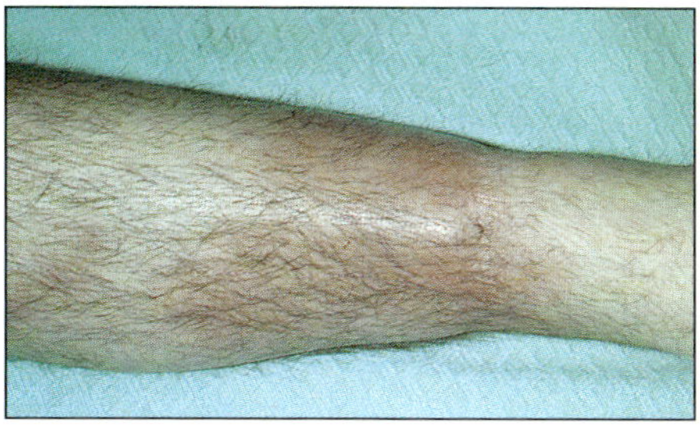

3 Erythema nodosum.

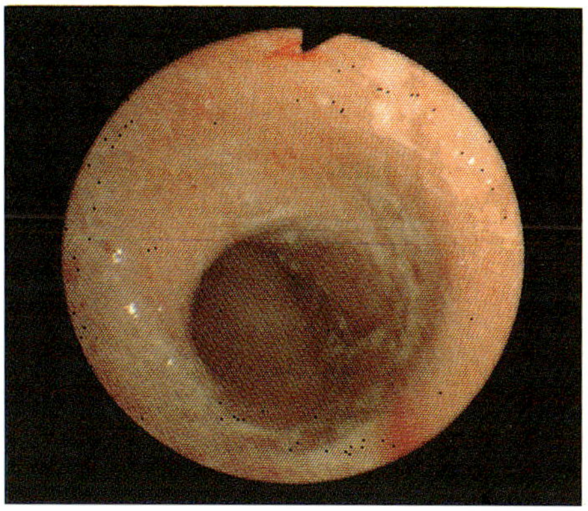

4

4 Sigmoidoscopic view.

Answers and comments

5 In any patient with an exacerbation of idiopathic inflammatory bowel disease it is essential to exclude an infective cause for their deterioration. These patients are no less likely than normal people to get enteropathic infections. This patient had in fact been given a course of antibiotics for his leg ulcer and it was important therefore to exclude Clostridium difficile causing pseudomembranous colitis. Stool culture and examination for Clostridium difficile toxin level are essential as is a sigmoidoscopy and biopsy. The sigmoidoscopic appearance is shown in **4** and the biopsy in **5**. Stool culture was negative and the biopsy confirmed active colitis.

5

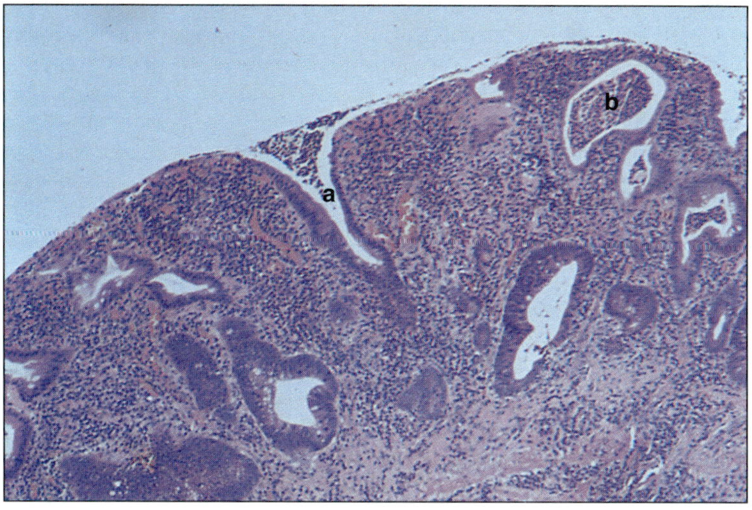

5 Rectal biopsy showing active colitis. The crypts (**a**) are short and irregular. There is goblet cell depletion and crypt abscesses (**b**) are present. A dense inflammatory infiltrate is seen in the mucosa.

6 The patient should receive a blood transfusion to raise his haemoglobin. Frequently severe colitics are hypokalaemic, but this was not the case in this patient. In view of the fact that the patient was systemically unwell, systemic steroids either orally or intravenously should be used. If there were no systemic upset and if the x-ray had suggested disease limited to the left colon, then rectal steroids might have sufficed. Salazopyrine or one of the newer non-sulpha containing 5 amino-salicylic acid derivatives should also be given, not only for its acute effects but also to start the patient on long-term prophylactic therapy. If treatment is clearly not working after a reasonable trial period, then an appropriate surgeon should be asked to see the patient with a view to surgical resection of the colon. The pyoderma gangrenosum cleared up with topical antibiotics and the use of steroids (**6**). The patient settled rapidly with oral steroids and salazopyrine and was able to gradually have the steroids withdrawn over the next 2 months. Once he had settled, a formal colonoscopic examination of the colon was undertaken and multiple biopsies obtained. Although most simply showed the changes of chronic ulcerative colitis, one biopsy showed additional changes (**7a** and **b**).

7 The indications for surgery are: a) for fulminant colitis which has not responded to treatment; b) for toxic megacolon developing during treatment; c) for perforation or torrential haemorrhage; d) chronic ill health due to the colitis, or failure of medical therapy; e) colonic cancer arising in ulcerative colitis and f) for persistent severe dysplasia.

Clinical progress

The patient was found to have severe dysplasia on biopsies taken from the caecum, as shown in **7a** and **b**. Colonoscopy was repeated after several months on two separate occasions and at each time severe dysplasia was demonstrated in the same area. The patient was counselled about these findings and decided to opt for elective surgery with a permanent ileostomy rather than for total colectomy with a pouch reconstruction and ileo-anal anastomosis. He has remained well ever since and has had no further dermatological problems.

6

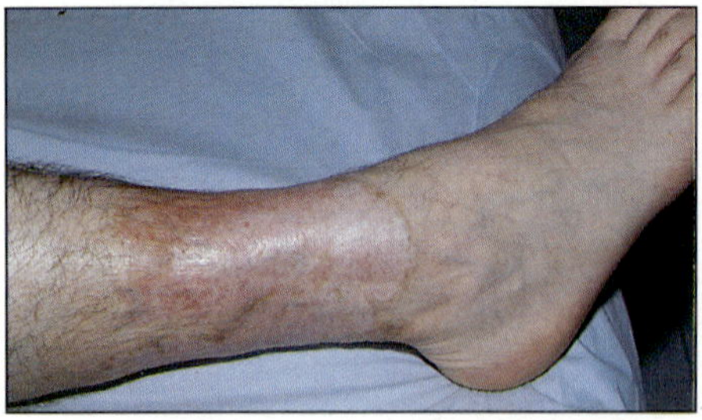

6 View of skin after use of antibiotics and steroids for pyoderma gangrenosum.

7a

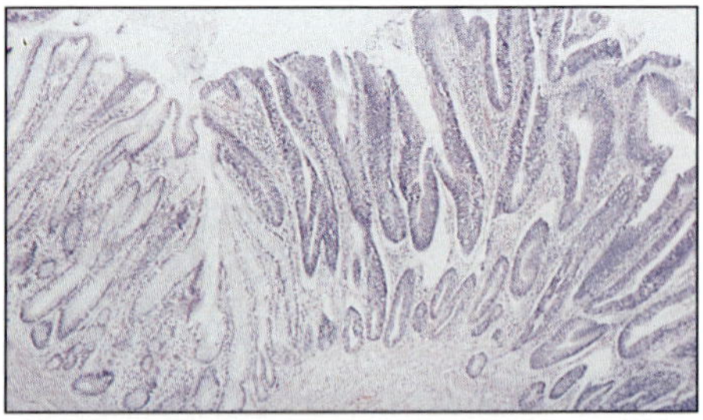

7b

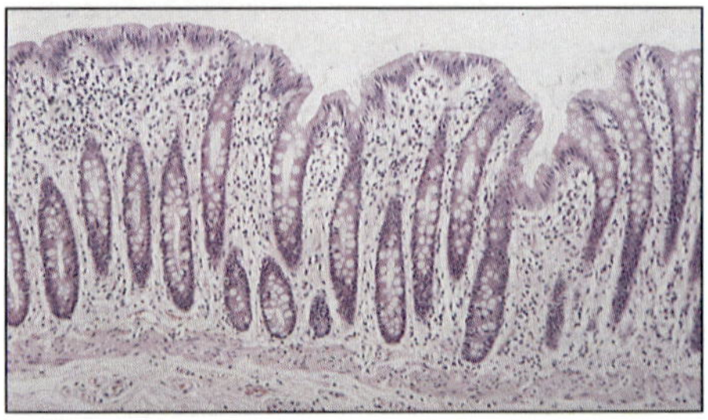

7a Dysplasia which is severe on the right side of the picture. **7b** Normal colonic mucosa for comparison.

Case 12

Tired and itching at 54

A mother of a junior hospital doctor was brought to the gastroenterology clinic. For over 6 months this pleasant business woman had grown increasingly tired, such that she no longer felt able to continue work. She would fall asleep on returning from work and even when awake was not as alert as she used to be. She had also become increasingly more forgetful, and was noted by her relatives to be mildly confused at times. Four weeks before attending the clinic she noted ankle swelling and mild abdominal distension. Pruritus had been present for a similar length of time and she was noted to be slightly jaundiced for 1 week preceding her visit. She never drank more than 12 units of alcohol per week and there was no family history of liver disease. On examination the patient was pigmented, but had recently been on holiday to Spain, and was mildly icteric. There were some spider naevi on her hands and arms and she had mild palmar erythema. Abdominal examination revealed moderate hepato-splenomegaly with some ascites. She had oedema to mid-calf level.

Investigations

Haematology and Biochemistry chart on page 52; Liver Biopsy (**1**).

1

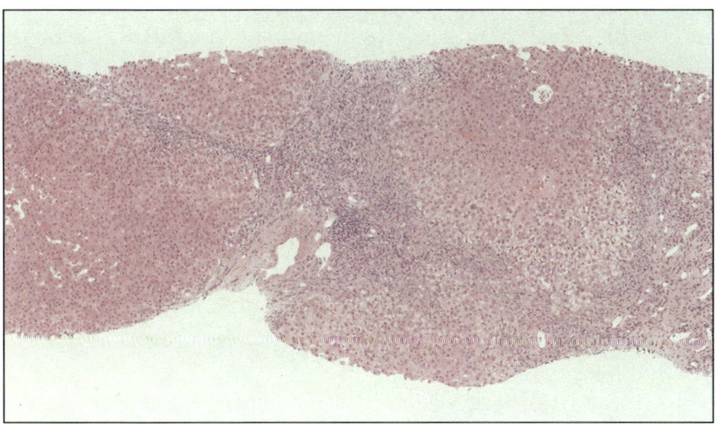

1 Liver biopsy.

Questions

1 What is the diagnosis ?
2 What further investigations are required ?
3 What does the liver biopsy show ?
4 What treatment would you offer initially ?
5 Her liver function tests 6 months later were: Bilirubin 23 μmol/l; Alk Phosph 124 U/l; ALT 28
What treatment do you think the patient has had?

Case 12

		Normal Range			Normal Range
Hb	12.6	11.5–16.0 **g/dl**	**MCHC**	33.9	33–36 **g/dl**
Hct	42.6	33–47 **%**	**Platelets**	69	150–400/ **10^9/l**
MCV	96.2	80–100 **fl**	**WCC**	6.7	3.5–11 **/ 10^9/l**
MCH	32.7	28–33 **pg**	**ESR**	22	< 20 **mm/hr**
Sodium	142	135–145 **mmol/l**	**Blood sugar**	3.8	3.5–7.2 **mmol/l**
Potassium	3.5	3.5–5.0 **mmol/l**	**Bilirubin**	84	2–17 **mmol/l**
Chloride	97	95–105 **mmol/l**	**Alk. Phos.**	1493	35–125 **U/l**
Bicarbonate	22	20–30 **mmol/l**	**ALT**	98	0–35 **U/l**
Urea	6.8	2.5–7.0 **mmol/l**	**GGT**	864	0–35 **U/l**
Creatinine	68	50–150 **mmol/l**	**Albumin**	23	36–52 **g/l**
Phosphate	0.73	0.7–1.4 **mmol/l**	**Globulin**	46	22–32 **g/l**
Calcium	2.18	2.2–2.6 **mmol/l**	**CRP**	44	5 **mg/l**
Prothrombin time		24 **sec**	**Control**		13 **sec**

Answers and Discussion

1 This patient is clearly suffering from decompensated cirrhosis. In a female of this age, who drank very little alcohol the most likely diagnosis is Primary Biliary Cirrhosis, although other forms of chronic liver disease need to be excluded. The presence of pigmentation would fit with the diagnosis of primary biliary cirrhosis, the other chronic liver disease associated with pigmentation being haemachromatosis. The pattern of liver function test abnormality with the very high alkaline phosphatase and GGT and mild elevation of ALT is typical of PBC.

2 First, investigation should be aimed at confirming the cause of the cirrhosis and second at ascertaining the reason for the recent decompensation. The causes of cirrhosis that need to be excluded are::

Hepatitis B and C:–HBsAg, HBcAb, HCAb
Auto-immune Chronic Active Hepatitis:– SMA, ANA.
Primary Biliary Cirrhosis:– AMA.
Alpha-1-antitrypsin deficiency:– alpha-1-antitrypsin level
Wilson's disease:– caeruloplasmin and copper levels
Haemachromatosis:–iron, iron binding capacity, % saturation and ferritin levels.

Decompensation in a cirrhotic patient can occur as a result of electrolyte imbalance, particularly hypokalaemia, infection, gastrointestinal bleeding, drug ingestion and development of hepatocellular carcinoma.

Investigation is thus aimed at excluding these conditions. A full blood count, electrolytes and alpha-fetoprotein should be measured and a full infection screen, including blood cultures and ascites culture, performed. The latter is important as Spontaneous Bacterial Peritonitis can be easily missed clinically. Ascitic fluid should be injected into blood-culture-medium bottles to increase the likelihood of a positive culture, because normally there are very few organisms per ml, and the chances of plating these by direct culture are more limited. A neutrophil count in the ascitic fluid if raised is also significant and suggests infection. A scan of the liver either by CT or ultrasound is essential to exclude a mass lesion. It must not be forgotten, however, that simple deterioration in hepatic function is also a common cause of liver failure with encephalopathy and fluid retention. This patient's AMA was positive with a titre of 1:512 , and her SMA was positive with a titre of 1:32. All other antibodies and investigations were negative, and no specific cause for her decompensation was evident other than progressive liver disease.

3 The liver biopsy shows established cirrhosis with few bile ducts and some chronic inflammatory cells. There is no evidence of hepatocellular carcinoma, which is uncommon in Primary Biliary Cirrhosis.

4 Initial treatment should be aimed at controlling her encephalopathy and restoring normal fluid balance. A low protein and low salt diet should be instituted, the former to reduce the encephalopathy, the latter to reduce fluid retention. Lactulose therapy with or without oral neomycin is used for the treatment of encephalopathy and in some units dietary supplementation with branch chain amino-acids is added. For mild degrees of fluid retention an aldosterone antagonist (spironolactone) is the first line of treatment of fluid retention, supplemented in more resistant cases by the addition of a small amount of loop diuretic such as frusemide. For those patients with marked ascites and oedema the modern line of treatment is to institute daily 2–4 litre paracenteses with replacement of lost protein by 20 gm salt free albumin, intravenously, for each litre of fluid removed. This has been shown to speed resolution of the ascites, shorten hospital stay and not increase the incidence of encephalopathy. In any patient with decompensated chronic liver disease consideration should be given to liver transplantation, and thus a full assessment of the patient made with that in mind.

5 Currently there is no specific drug treatment for PBC that would normalise liver function. Figure **2** shows the patient a few months after orthotopic liver transplantation. Primary biliary cirrhosis is one of the main indications for liver transplantation for chronic liver disease. Primary sclerosing cholangitis is also a common indication. Most other causes of cirrhosis of a non-infectious type can be transplanted including stable abstinent alcoholic cirrhotics. Figure **3** shows the explant liver from another patient with chronic Hepatitis B. The liver shows a typical macronodular cirrhosis.

2

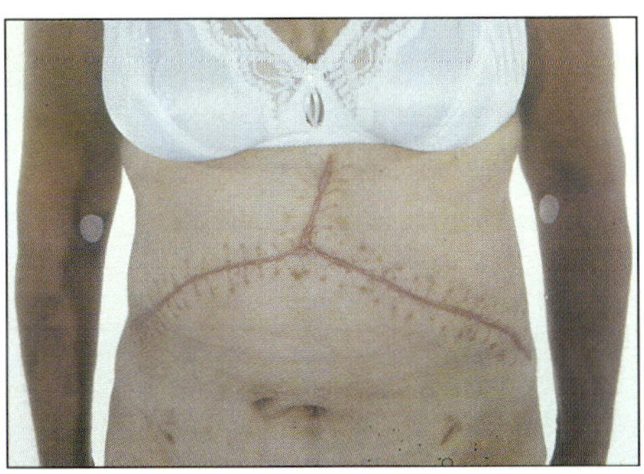

2 Post liver transplant scar.

3

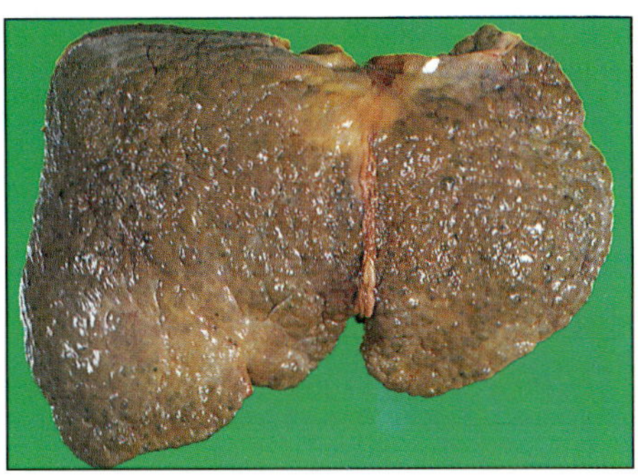

3 Explant liver from another patient.

Case 13

Elderly man with diarrhoea

This 76-year-old man was referred from his local hospital with a 4-year history of diarrhoea. The diarrhoea was intermittent and sometimes was explosive in nature, splattering into the pan with much flatus and having a foul smell. He had lost several pounds in weight. On investigation in the other hospital no apparent cause for the diarrhoea had been found apart from diverticular disease. He was noted to have a low vitamin B_{12} level, although no explanation for this had been sought. On examination there was no significant abnormality found.

Investigations

Haematology and Biochemistry chart on page 55; Radiology: Barium enema (**1**).

1

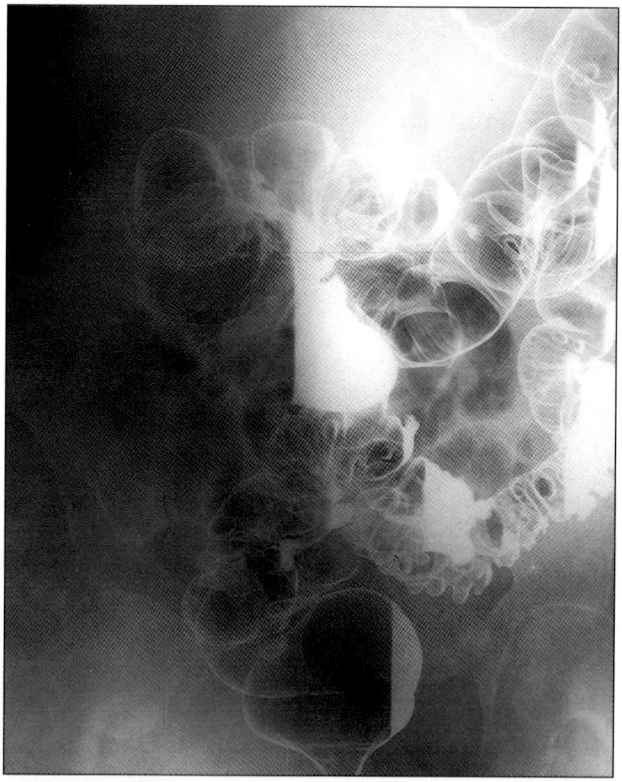

1 Barium enema.

Questions

1 What do the above results suggest?
2 What investigations would be appropriate next?
3 What is the relevance of the barium enema findings?

		Normal Range			Normal Range
Hb	13.8	12.5–18 **g/dl**	**MCHC**	34.9	33–36 **g/dl**
Hct	39.5	33–47 **%**	**Platelets**	306	150–400/ **10^9/l**
MCV	86.7	80–100 **fl**	**WCC**	9.9	3.5–11 **/ 10^9/l**
MCH	30.3	28–33 **pg**	**ESR**	9	< 20 **mm/hr**
Sodium	141	135–145 **mmol/l**	**Blood sugar**	5.3	3.5–7.2 **mmol/l**
Potassium	3.7	3.5–5.0 **mmol/l**	**Bilirubin**	7	2–17 **mmol/l**
Chloride	102	95–105 **mmol/l**	**Alk. Phos.**	56	35–125 **U/l**
Bicarbonate	25	20–30 **mmol/l**	**ALT**	15	0–35 **U/l**
Urea	3.3	2.5–7.0 **mmol/l**	**GGT**	13	0–35 **U/l**
Creatinine	82	50–150 **mmol/l**	**Albumin**	37	36–52 **g/l**
Phosphate	0.66	0.7–1.4 **mmol/l**	**Globulin**	27	22–32 **g/l**
Calcium	2.06	2.2–2.6 **mmol/l**	**CRP**	<5	<5 **mg/l**
Serum folate	7.8	1.5–5.5 **µg/l**			
Serum B_{12}	108	170–590 **µg/l**			

Answers and discussion

1 The positive findings are a low-serum calcium, low B_{12} and rather high-serum folate. In the presence of a history as outlined above malabsorption should be considered. It is not unusual to find that the haemoglobin is not lowered in the early stages of malabsorption.

2 There are two approaches to the further investigation of the above patient. The traditional way would be to first prove the diagnosis of malabsorption and then to investigate the mechanism concerned and the underlying cause. This approach would involve some method of assessing fat malabsorption such as 3-day faecal fat collection, and in many centres this is only undertaken when there is little clue to the cause of diarrhoea in a problem patient. If on clinical grounds and in the light of preliminary investigation malabsorption is suspected, a more direct approach to investigation is usually undertaken. The basis of this is to ascertain whether there is macroscopic structural abnormality in the small bowel (such as Crohn's disease, fistulae, blind loops, diverticulae or abnormal motility), microscopic abnormality of the mucosa (coeliac, Whipple's disease, lymphangiectasia) or whether there is pancreatic or hepatic abnormalities. This simple division of the causes of malabsorption will rapidly bring to light the commoner causes.The next most important investigations would be a small bowel biopsy, small bowel radiology and a pancreatic scan, either CT or ultrasound.

3 The sigmoid diverticular disease is not relevant in the diagnosis of malabsorption and is rarely the cause of diarrhoea. In patients presenting with diarrhoea, after rectal examination and sigmoidoscopy a barium enema is a reasonable next investigation.

Further investigations

1 Small bowel biopsy (**2**).
2 Small bowel barium follow through examination (**3**).
3 CT scan of pancreas (**4**).

Questions

4 What does the small bowel biopsy show?
5 What abnormality is shown on the barium study ?
6 Is the pancreas normal on the CT scan?

2

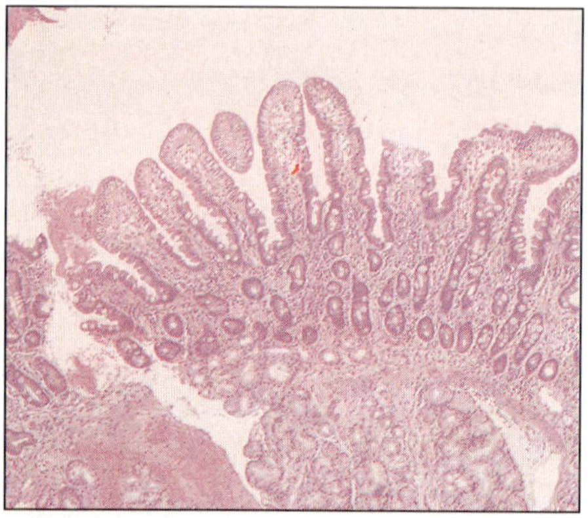

2 Small bowel biopsy.

3a

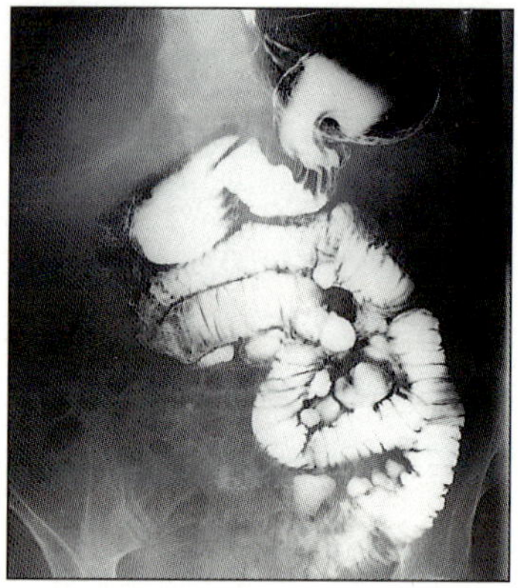

3b

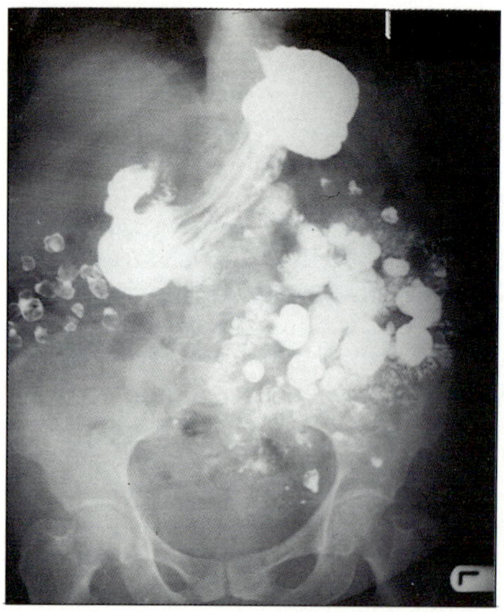

3 a, b Barium follow through.

4

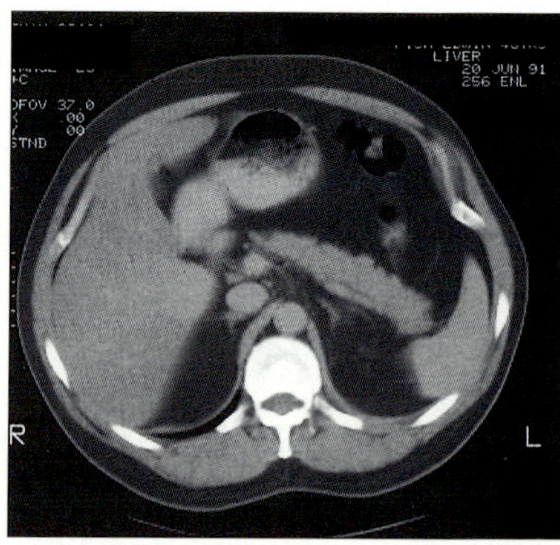

4 CT scan of pancreas.

Answers and discussion

4 The small bowel biopsy is entirely normal with slender finger-like villi with no increase in inflammatory cells.
5 There are numerous small-bowel diverticulae filled with barium.

6 The pancreas is entirely normal with no evidence of calcification, cysts or either atrophy or enlargement. This patient thus has evidence of small bowel diverticulae with malabsorption.

Questions

7 What is the mechanism of malabsorption in these patients?
8 How would you confirm this ?
9 What treatment would you give this patient?

Answers and discussion

7 The mechanism is thought to be due to bacterial overgrowth within the diverticulae. The bacteria can then split or deconjugate the bile salts rendering them less soluble and thus decreasing fat absorption by reducing the concentration of bile salts to below the critical micellar concentration. Some bacteria dehydrogenate the bile salts again rendering them less soluble. The unabsorbed fat may then undergo rancidification which will contribute to diarrhoea. The high bacterial content of the bowel may use up intraluminal B_{12} so resulting in reduced levels available for absorption. It is not uncommon for high levels of folate to be generated by these bacteria.
8 There are three methods of confirming small-bowel bacterial overgrowth. The gold standard, least often performed, and least pleasant for the patient is small-bowel aspiration with samples collected by a fine bore sterile tube swallowed by the patient. This was often performed at the same time as small-bowel biopsy. Anaerobic as well as aerobic cultures are required.

The other methods use breath tests. The breath hydrogen test depends upon the splitting of either dextrose or lactulose by excess small-bowel bacteria to produce hydrogen. This diffuses across the mucosa into the blood and is taken to the lungs where it equilibrates with alveolar air and is exhaled in the breath. Samples of end expiratory air are collected from the mouthpiece end of a Haldane tube, and are injected into a hydrogen gas analyser (**5** and **6**). A rise in breath hydrogen shortly after ingestion of the substrate sugar is taken to signify bacterial overgrowth.

The second type of breath test depends upon the ability of the bacteria to deconjugate a radioactively labelled bile salt. The glycine is labelled with C^{14} and is attached to cholic acid. The labelled, conjugated bile salt is given as a drink

5

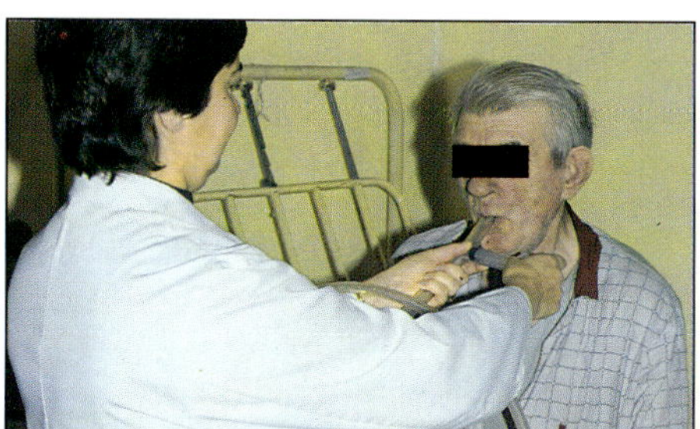

5 Collecting expired gas using a Haldane tube.

6

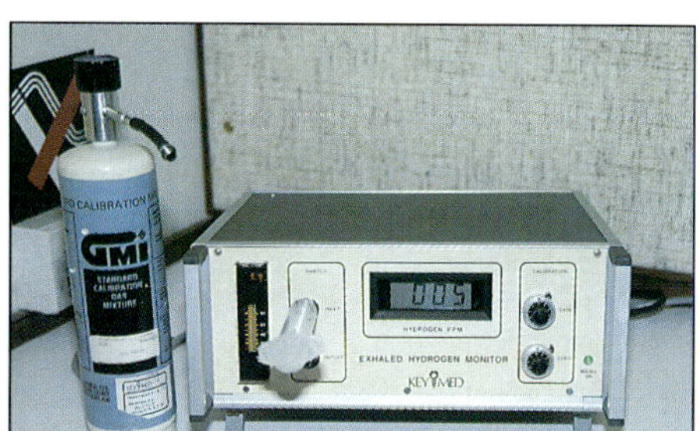

6 Hydrogen gas analyser.

and at regular intervals the patient is asked to breathe into a CO_2 trapping solution mixed with a scintillation fluid that can be counted in a liquid scintillation counter. If excess bacteria are present, and these are capable of deconjugation, the labelled glycine will be split from the cholic acid, the glycine absorbed and metabolised with the production of labelled carbon dioxide. This is then exhaled in the breath, trapped in the scintillation fluid and counted. It is said that the combination of the two breath tests will pick up all of the bacterial overgrowth patients found by direct aspiration and culture. This patient's breath hydrogen test is shown in **7**.

7

TIME	HYDROGEN CONCENTRATION
8.30	0–2
	0–2
	0–2
8.35	75 g Dextrose
8.45	4
8.50	12
9.05	27
9.20	43
9.35	51
9.50	63
10.05	67
10.20	70
10.35	65
10.50	47
11.05	33

7 Results of patient's breath hydrogen test.

9 Treatment of bacterial overgrowth may take several forms. If there is a correctable anatomical abnormality that predisposes to the overgrowth such as a fistula, then consideration should be given to its surgical correction. In many patients, as in this one, surgery would not be possible because of the extensive nature of the condition. In this case use of antibiotics is usually effective. The commonly used antibiotics are oxytetracycline, metronidazole or occasionally lincomycin or ciprofloxacin. These can be given either in defined courses, with further courses only administered on return of symptoms, or as continuous treatment for those who relapse frequently. Some gastroenterologists use alternating courses of oxytetracycline and metronidazole.

This patient had a dramatic response to oxytetracycline 250 mg t.d.s., but relapsed shortly after completing a 4-week course. He has now been on continuous treatment for 4 years with no further symptomatic relapse.

Case 14

Weight loss in a 20 year old

A consultant radiologist referred a 20-year-old Irish radiographer who had been losing weight for several months. She had lost a total of 10 kg in weight and was finding it difficult to perform her duties because of frequent bowel movements. She felt tired and listless and had recently developed ankle swelling. On examination she looked pale, had mild pitting ankle oedema and had clearly lost weight.

Investigations

Haematology and Biochemistry chart on page 60; Radiology: Chest x-ray: normal; Small-bowel barium follow through(**1**); (performed by the radiologist before referral).

1

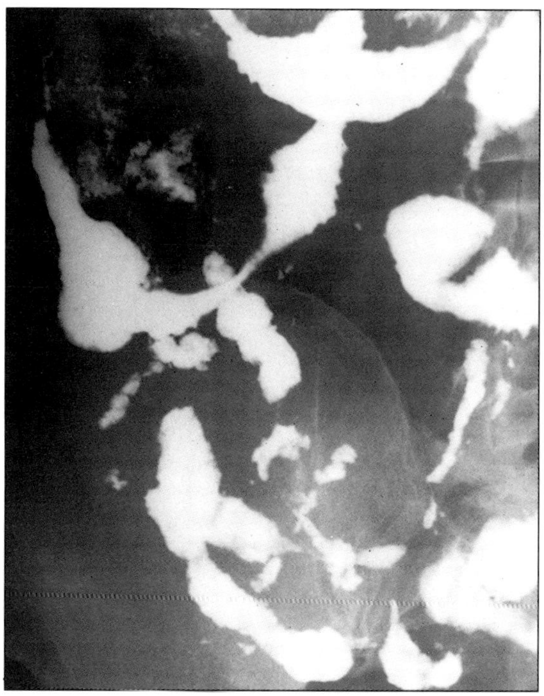

1 Small bowel barium follow through.

Questions

1 What do the investigations demonstrate?
2 What is the differential diagnosis?
3 What is the relevance of her nationality and what further questions should you ask?
4 What investigations should be performed?
5 What treatment would you advise?

		Normal Range			Normal Range
Hb	9.6	11.5–16.0 **g/dl**	**MCHC**	34.8	33–36 **g/dl**
Hct	27.7	33–47 **%**	**Platelets**	344	150–400/ **10^9/l**
MCV	108	80–100 **fl**	**WCC**	5.6	3.5–11 **/ 10^9/l**
MCH	36.5	28–33 **pg**	**ESR**	15	< 20 **mm/hr**
Sodium	144	135–145 **mmol/l**	**Blood sugar**	5.0	3.5–7.2 **mmol/l**
Potassium	14.3	3.5–5.0 **mmol/l**	**Bilirubin**	5	2–17 **mmol/l**
Chloride	106	95–105 **mmol/l**	**Alk. Phos.**	85	35–125 **U/l**
Bicarbonate	24	20–30 **mmol/l**	**ALT**	12	0–35 **U/l**
Urea	5.8	2.5–7.0 **mmol/l**	**GGT**	15	0–35 **U/l**
Creatinine	67	50–150 **mmol/l**	**Albumin**	28	36–52 **g/l**
Phosphate	0.80	0.7–1.4 **mmol/l**	**Globulin**	26	22–32 **g/l**
Calcium	2.13	2.2–2.6 **mmol/l**	**CRP**	5	<5 **mg/l**
Serum folate	1.3	1.5–5.5 **μg/l**			
B_{12}	167	170–590 **μg/l**			
Ferritin	43	17–165 **μg/l**			

Answers and discussion

1 The patient has a macrocytic anaemia with a low folate and low ferritin. The B_{12} is at the lower end of the normal range. In addition both the albumin and calcium are low. These results suggest malabsorption. The barium follow through shows flocculation of barium with slightly dilated loops of jejunum but no other abnormality. The appearance was said to be consistent with malabsorption but not diagnostic.

2 The differential diagnosis lies between coeliac disease and Crohn's disease as the two common causes of malabsorption in the UK. Giardiasis would be another possibility.

3 Coeliac disease is particularly common in patients who come from the west coast of Ireland and thus she should be asked whether her family comes from the Galway area, which has the highest rate of coeliac disease in the world. The frequency of this condition in this area is approximately 1:200, whereas in the rest of the UK it is 1:2000.

4 To prove the diagnosis of coeliac disease a small-bowel biopsy should be undertaken. If the mucosa demonstrates the characteristic abnormality, then the patient should be treated and most would advise a repeat biopsy to be performed after 4–6 months. Some experts recommend a 'Gluten Challenge' and a repeat biopsy, although in most clinical practices this is not undertaken. The small bowel biopsy can either be obtained using a Crosby Capsule (**2a** and **b**) or via biopsies taken through a standard gastroscope inserted far down the duodenum. If the latter route is used then 4 biopsies are thought to be required.

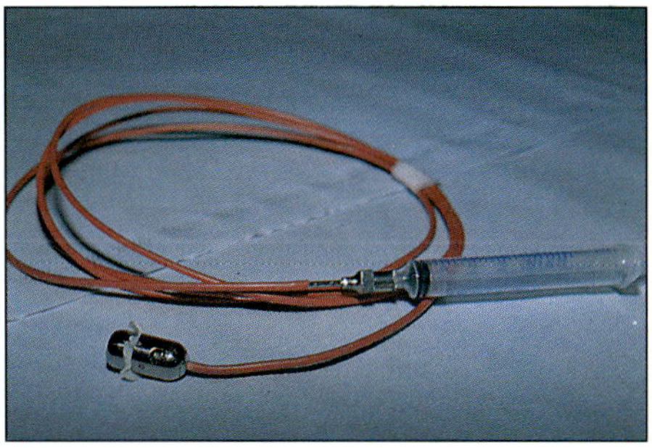
2a Crosby capsule.

Before any biopsy a check must be made of the patient's clotting and a platelet count and prothrombin time measured. The prothrombin time is particularly important, because if there is significant fat malabsorption, vitamin K may be malabsorbed with consequent prolongation of the prothrombin time and the risk of bleeding. In some units screening tests for coeliac disease may be used such as anti-reticulin antibodies and anti-gliadin antibodies. Tests of intestinal permeability (differential sugar absorption with cellobiose and mannitol or lactulose and mannitol) are also used by some as screening tests but have not become widely used since the change to gastroscopic small-bowel biopsy. The use of this means of biopsy is rapid, without need for screening (c.f. Crosby capsule) and reliably provides tissue. On many occasions the capsules would either not fire or no adequate sample would be obtained. If biopsies do not show evidence of coeliac disease or giardiasis, then the next step would be to arrange a contrast study of the small intestine to look for Crohn's disease.

5 If the biopsies are consistent with coeliac disease, then the patient should have the nature of the disease explained and should be referred to a dietitian to start on a gluten-free diet. The patient should be advised to join the National Coeliac Society who provide updated lists of gluten-containing foods. If the patient is short of vitamins, iron or is anaemic, it is often helpful to give the appropriate supplements while waiting for the diet to work.

Investigations

Histopathology: Small bowel biopsy (**3**).

Question

6 What abnormalities are shown on this patient's small bowel biopsy and are these changes consistent with coeliac disease?

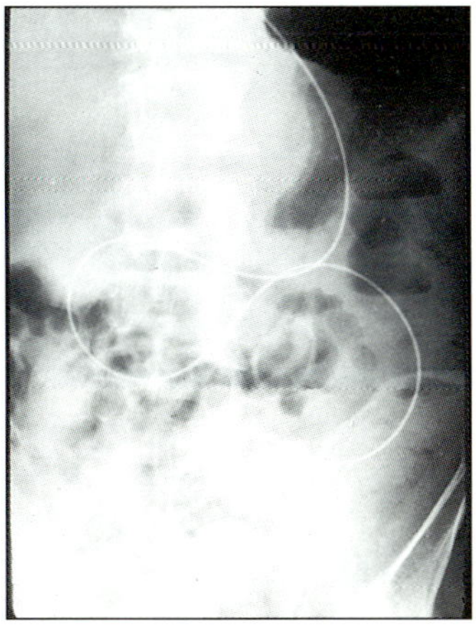

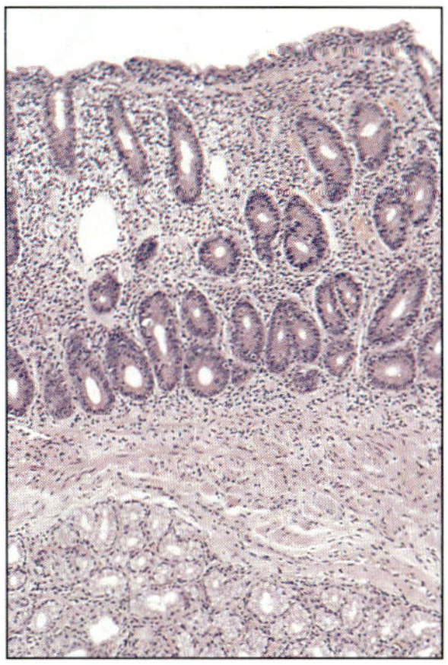

2b Capsule *in situ* in the jejunum.
3 Histopathology of small bowel biopsy.

Answer and discussion

6 The biopsy shows small, stunted villi with a dense inflammatory infiltrate, intraepithelial lymphocytes and crypt hyperplasia. These are the classical changes of coeliac disease and can be compared with the repeat biopsy (**4**) performed some 6 months later, the patient having been on a gluten-free diet. On this biopsy the mucosa has returned to normal with fine finger like villi. Figures **5a** and **b** show the appearances seen under a dissecting microscope.

4

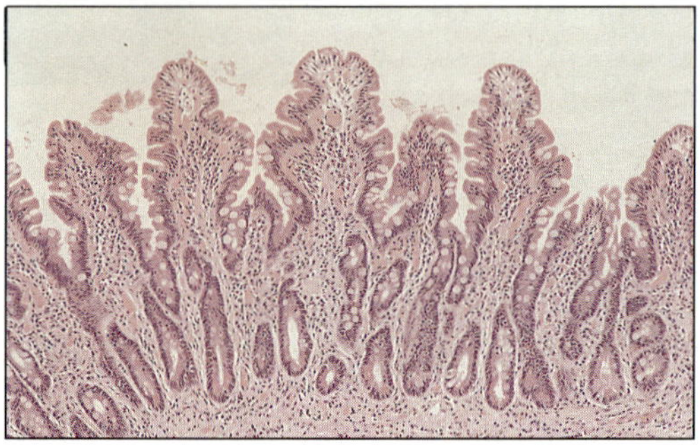

4 Histopathology of a repeat biopsy.

5a

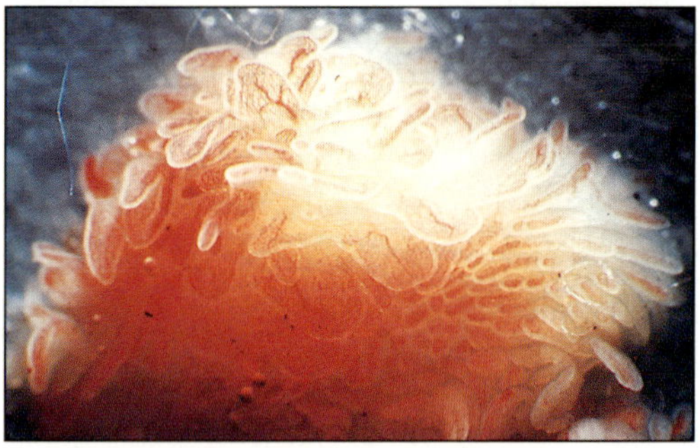

5 Jejunal mucosa seen with the dissecting microscope: (**a**) normal; (**b**) villous atrophy.

5b

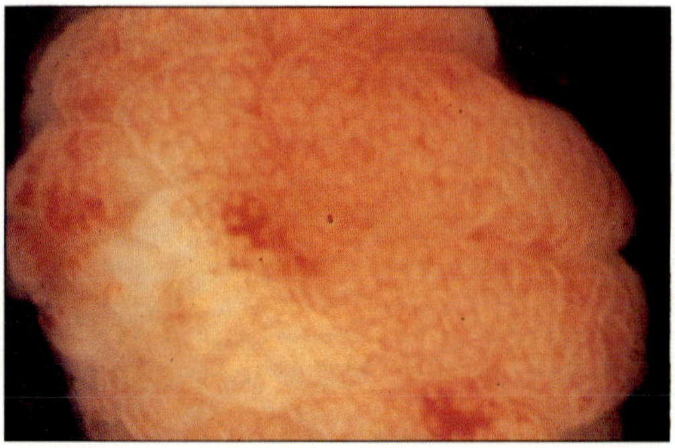

Case 15

Abdominal pain and diarrhoea

A 24-year-old student was admitted twice to a local small hospital with colicky right iliac fossa pain, vomiting, anorexia and weight loss. These admissions were within 2 months of each other and the symptoms resolved rapidly with nil by mouth, intravenous fluids and pethidine for pain. Between these attacks which lasted 1 week, the patient had mild right iliac fossa discomfort, some looseness of stools and 4 bowel movements per day instead of her usual 1 motion. She had similar but milder symptoms for about 4 months prior to the first attack, with recurrent apthoid mouth ulcers. She had lost about 7 kg in weight and was tired and depressed. Investigations in the local hospital were said to be normal. She was referred for a second opinion in view of the lack of progress.The only additional history was that her aunt had coeliac disease.

Investigations

Haematology and Biochemistry chart on page 64. Straight x-ray (**1**).

1

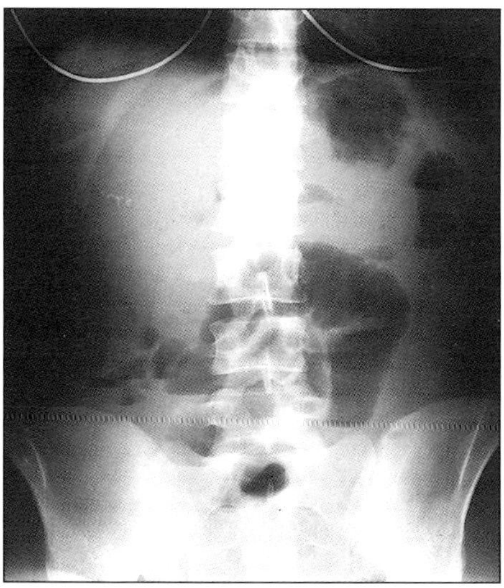

1 Plain abdominal x-ray (erect).

2

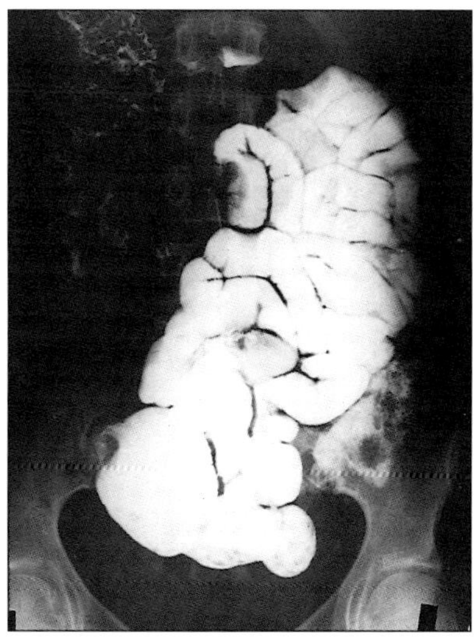

2 Barium follow through.

Questions

1 What is the differential diagnosis?
2 What does the straight x-ray show?
3 What further investigations would you undertake?

		Normal Range			Normal Range
Hb	10.8	11.5–16.0 **g/dl**	**MCHC**	35.2	33–36 **g/dl**
Hct	32.1	33–47 **%**	**Platelets**	535	150–400/ **10^9/l**
MCV	76.0	80–100 **fl**	**WCC**	10.1	3.5–11 **/ 10^9/l**
MCH	27.1	28–33 **pg**	**ESR**	34	< 20 **mm/hr**
Sodium	144	135–145 **mmol/l**	**Blood sugar**	3.9	3.5–7.2 **mmol/l**
Potassium	4.6	3.5–5.0 **mmol/l**	**Bilirubin**	4	2–17 **mmol/l**
Chloride	100	95–105 **mmol/l**	**Alk. Phos.**	39	35–125 **U/l**
Bicarbonate	23	20–30 **mmol/l**	**ALT**	18	0–35 **U/l**
Urea	3.3	2.5–7.0 **mmol/l**	**GGT**	16	0–35 **U/l**
Creatinine	78	50–150 **mmol/l**	**Albumin**	38	36–52 **g/l**
Phosphate	0.92	0.7–1.4 **mmol/l**	**Globulin**	26	22–32 **g/l**
Calcium	2.03	2.2–2.6 **mmol/l**	**CRP**	26	<5 **mg/l**

Answers and discussion

1 In the UK the likely diagnosis is either an Irritable Bowel Syndrome, Coeliac disease or terminal ileal Crohn's disease. In an Asian population tuberculosis would be a possibility. There are other much less common disorders affecting the terminal small bowel such as actinomycosis or small- bowel tumours. In view of her family history of coeliac disease, ulcerative jejunoilietis as a complication of coeliac disease must be considered.
2 The x-ray shows a few fluid levels and distended small-bowel loops in the lower abdomen. This finding, together with the slightly raised ESR and CRP and the mild degree of anaemia, suggests the presence of organic disease rather than an irritable bowel syndrome.
3 The most important investigation would be radiology of the small bowel and possibly a small intestinal biopsy. She already had had a barium meal and follow-through examination at the local hospital but this had been reported as normal. On review of the films an abnormality was seen (**2**).

Questions

4 What does the repeat barium study show (**2**)?
5 What further studies would you undertake?

Answers and discussion

4 A dilated loop of ileum is present, with the suggestion of a narrowed area distal to the dilated segment. Mucosal detail is not good. Repeat pictures obtained revealed obvious Crohn's disease affecting the terminal ileum (**3**). In view of her history of diarrhoea, it would be reasonable to undertake sigmoidoscopy and biopsy to look for evidence of colonic involvement. However, full colonic assessment could only be achieved by either barium enema examination or full colonoscopy. The latter is a better investigation because it does not involve

further radiology and will permit biopsies to be taken from around the colon and possibly from the terminal ileum, which might provide histological proof of the diagnosis. It is all too easy to forget just how many x-rays young patients are subjected to in the lifetime of a chronic disease such as Crohn's.

5 Another useful way of assessing the extent of inflammatory bowel disease is to use isotopically labelled white cells and to scan the abdomen to look at their localisation. Either Indium or Technetium can be used. Typical scans showing colonic and ileal disease are shown in **4**. In this patient colonoscopy failed to show any evidence of colonic disease either macroscopically or on biopsy. Isotope studies were not carried out in view of the diagnostic barium studies. A full nutritional assessment should be undertaken, including assessment for iron, folate or B_{12} deficiency.

3

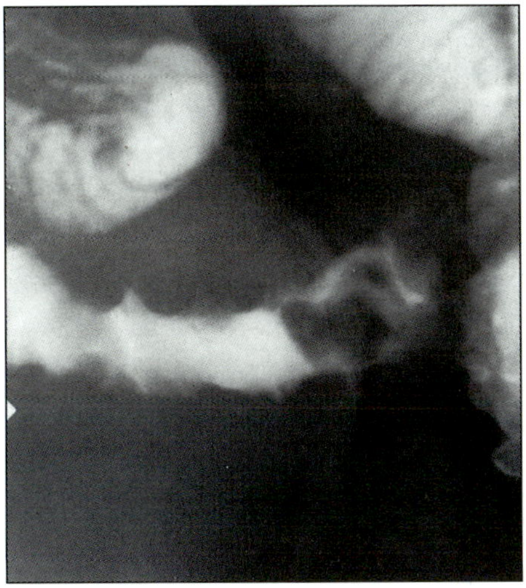

3 Part of the small bowel X-ray showing an area of terminal ileum with stricture formation and 'rose-thorn' ulceration.

4

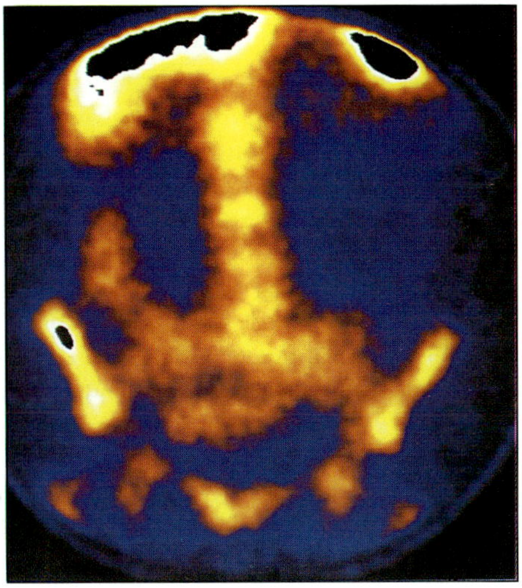

4 Scan showing colonic and ileal disease.

Questions

6 What are the causes of diarrhoea in Crohn's disease?
7 What treatment would you consider for this patient?

Answers and Discussion

6 There are several different causes for diarrhoea in Crohn's disease. Colonic Crohn's disease can cause diarrhoea due to the inflammation and ulceration of the mucosa if the bowel is actively inflamed, but can cause frequent need for defaecation because of thickening and fibrosis of the wall of the colon with loss of compliance. In small bowel disease diarrhoea may be caused by bacterial overgrowth above strictures, secondary to fistulation between loops of bowel (**5**) and by involvement of the terminal ileum with secondary bile salt malabsorption and resulting choloretic diarrhoea. This is due to the unabsorbed bile salts irritating and causing secretory colonic diarrhoea.

Case 15

5

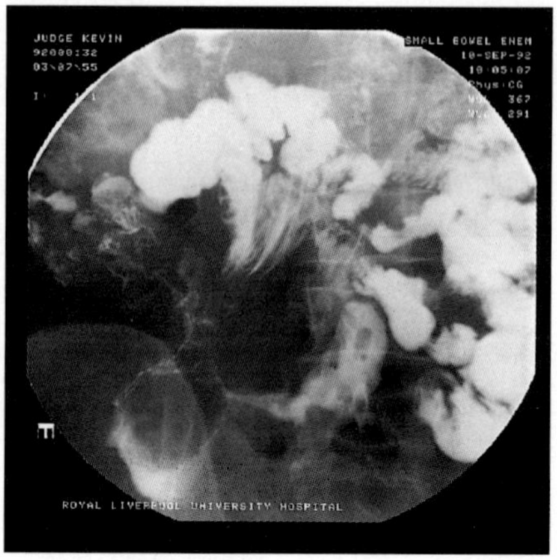

5 Bowel loop fistulation.

Active small bowel inflammation with Crohn's disease presumably also causes diarrhoea by a combination of the above as well as by secretion from the inflamed bowel. Small bowel to large bowel fistulae can also cause diarrhoea as can small bowel resection. If a large portion of the small bowel is resected, then the patient may suffer from the short bowel syndrome; terminal ileal resection alone can also cause diarrhoea by removing the absorptive site for bile salts and thus giving rise to choloretic diarrhoea. It is important to define the cause of diarrhoea in a patient with Crohn's disease in order to target treatment better.

7 This patient's predominant symptoms were of abdominal pain with partial small bowel obstruction, not the diarrhoea. Three main types of treatment exist for acute Crohn's, systemic steroids, enteral feeding with a liquid elemental or polymeric diet, or surgery. Surgery would be indicated for those patients who did not settle with medical therapy or where there was continuing small bowel obstruction. The choice for initial treatment between dietary management or steroids is a matter of preference and debate. Some studies show that elemental diet controls acute Crohn's as well as steroids, but there is considerable debate as to whether polymeric (protein hydrolysate, or peptide based) diets are as effective as elemental (amino-acid) based ones. Because of her initial severe symptoms with vomiting as a component, intravenous steroids were started. Initially her symptoms settled quickly. The initial intravenous fluids were replaced by an oral elemental diet, which tastes unpleasant and is often administered via a fine bore feeding tube. She managed to drink the diet provided it was kept cold. Steroids were continued but her abdominal pain returned within a few days of starting oral feeding and disappeared rapidly with fasting and intravenous fluids. It proved impossible to control her symptoms adequately with medical treatment and a surgeon was asked to see her.

Questions

8 What surgical options are there in the treatment of this patient?
9 What does the resected specimen (**6**) show ?
10 What specific complications are associated with terminal ileal resection ?

6
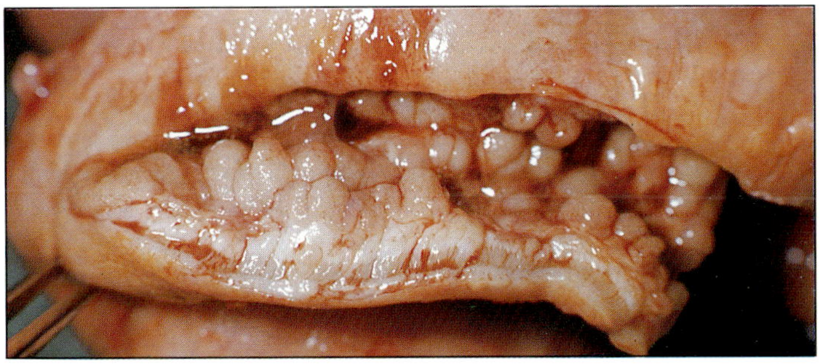

6 Part of resected ileum incised to show mucosal appearance.

Answers and discussion

8 Although resection of the involved portion of terminal ileum either at open operation or by laparoscopically assisted surgery is the mainstay of treatment, in those patients with a localised stricture, stricturoplasty is an alternative if the stricture is short or there are multiple short strictures. The use of this procedure avoids resection and thus loss of bowel length.
9 The specimen shows the typical appearances of Crohn's disease with linear ulceration, producing a cobblestone appearance. There is oedema and fibrotic thickenning of the intestinal wall.
10 Resection of the terminal ileum may result in both bile acid malabsorption with resulting fat malabsorption and choloretic diarrhoea as well as vitamin B_{12} malabsorption. Whether there is clinically significant malabsorption will depend on the extent of the resection and the health of the remaining ileum. If the ileocaecal valve is resected, there may be an increased risk of small-bowel bacterial overgrowth. Many gastroenterologists routinely prescribe regular injections of B_{12} to prevent the development of macrocytic anaemia. This patient had a laparoscopically assisted resection of her terminal ileum and caecum and was able to be discharged on the third postoperative day. Since that time she has had no symptoms at all and has not required any other medication. She is under long-term follow-up.

Case 16

Severe watery diarrhoea in a nurse

A 21-year-old nurse presented to her own hospital with a 6-month history of watery diarrhoea and weight loss of a couple of kilograms. There was no preceding history of note and she was engaged to be married and had just completed her qualifying examinations successfully. Physical examination was uninformative. She had not seen any blood in her stools, nor had she had any abdominal pain. The local gastroenterologist had undertaken several investigations delineated below.

Investigations

Haematology and Biochemistry chart below; Sigmoidoscopy (**1a** and **b**). Small bowel and large bowel radiology—negative

		Normal Range			Normal Range
Hb	13.1	11.5–16.0 **g/dl**	**MCHC**	33.3	33–36 **g/dl**
Hct	39.4	33–47 %	**Platelets**	313	150–400/ **10^9/l**
MCV	95.9	80–100 **fl**	**WCC**	5.0	3.5–11 **/ 10^9/l**
MCH	32.0	28–33 **pg**	**ESR**	12	< 20 **mm/hr**
Sodium	142	135–145 **mmol/l**	**Blood sugar**	3.6	3.5–7.2 **mmol/l**
Potassium	4.1	3.5–5.0 **mmol/l**	**Bilirubin**	10	2–17 **mmol/l**
Chloride	105	95–105 **mmol/l**	**Alk. Phos.**	77	35–125 **U/l**
Bicarbonate	23	20–30 **mmol/l**	**ALT**	23	0–35 **U/l**
Urea	5.1	2.5–7.0 **mmol/l**	**GGT**	12	0–35 **U/l**
Creatinine	83	50–150 **mmol/l**	**Albumin**	41	36–52 **g/l**
Phosphate	0.73	0.7–1.4 **mmol/l**	**Globulin**	25	22–32 **g/l**
Calcium	2.30	2.2–2.6 **mmol/l**	**CRP**	<5	<5 **mg/l**

Questions

1 What does the sigmoidoscopy show ?
2 What further initial investigation should be undertaken?
3 What are the two main pathophysiological types of diarrhoea?

Answers and discussion

1 The mucosa shows a normal vascular pattern without any evidence of hyperaemia, oedema, granularity or contact bleeding.
2 It is always important to look for infective or parasitic causes of chronic diarrhoea. Most enteric bacterial infections would not last for such a prolonged period; however, parasitic or protozoal infections need to be excluded. Giar-

1a 1b

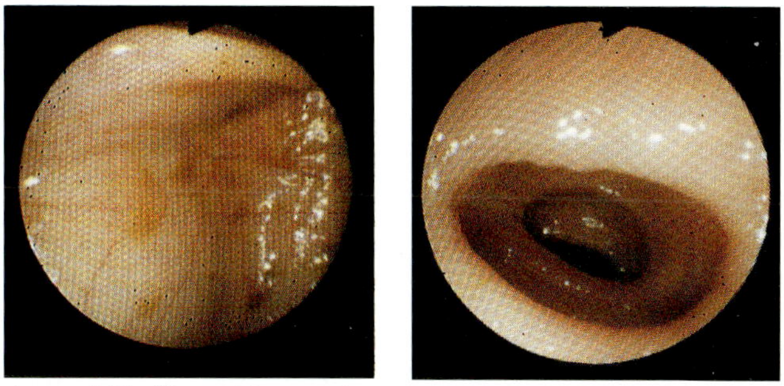

1a and **1b** Sigmoidoscopies.

diasis is particularly common and may present as either diarrhoea or as a malabsorptive picture.The increased number of patients with HIV infection and AIDS also often present to gastroenterologists with diarrhoea secondary to protozoal infection. It would thus be important to examine the faeces for ova, cysts and parasites as well as sending it for routine culture. If there is any history to suggest that the patient might have HIV infection, then after appropriate counselling, and with the patient's permission, blood should be sent for HIV testing. Another common condition often presenting with diarrhoea is coeliac disease. The patient should thus have a small-bowel biopsy, which can also be examined for parasites.

3 If all the above tests are normal, it is sensible to try and determine what sort of watery diarrhoea the patient is suffering from. There are basically two pathophysiological types – osmotic or secretory, and the further investigation of the patient can be divided into the investigation of these two categories. Before this is undertaken it is advisable to measure the stool volume, and this is quite easily done by measuring a 24-hour stool weight. Any weight less than 300 gm is classified as low-volume diarrhoea and may represent a local colonic cause, or poor rectal compliance and inability to retain small volumes of stool. Values over 600 gm per 24 hours are clearly elevated and further investigation is likely to reveal the underlying cause. Intermediate values should probably still be investigated, whereas low-volume diarrhoea is unlikely to need extensive further investigations. It is also very important to look at the collection,because very often a patient's idea of diarrhoea and a doctor's differ. A patient may mean an increased stool frequency rather than a change in consistency when talking about diarrhoea.

Questions

4 What are the two main methods of distinguishing osmotic from secretory diarrhoea?

5 Which of the two stool charts shown in **2** is typical of a secretory diarrhoea's response to fasting?

6 What are the common causes of an osmotic diarrhoea?

7 Which set of stool biochemical results shown in **3** correspond to a secretory diarrhoea?

8 What investigation has been carried out on this patient's urine (**4**) and what does it suggest as a cause for her diarrhoea?

9 What are the causes of a secretory diarrhoea?

Answers and discussion

4 The first method of value in distinguishing between these types of diarrhoea is the stool volume or weight response to total fasting. The patient has three consecutive 24-hour stool weights determined and these sent to the laboratory for faecal fat estimation, so helping to exclude occult malabsorption. The patient is then fasted for 72 hours while intravenous fluids are administered and faecal weights are measured for each day. If there is a fall in stool weight during the fast, this suggests an osmotic cause for the diarrhoea. Should the stool weight remain unchanged, a secretory diarrhoea is more likely. It is sensible to send the stools to the laboratory to have their osmolality, sodium and potassium concentration checked, particularly if the stool volume decreases. Measurements of faecal magnesium levels may also help.

The second test is to send a faecal sample to the laboratory to check the osmolality, sodium and potassium concentration. Normally the osmolality of a faecal fluid sample should is nearly the same as twice the sum of the sample's sodium and potassium concentrations. If there is an osmolar gap (the faecal osmolality is greater than twice the sum of their combined concentrations), this suggests the presence of another osmotically active substance. If the osmolality is lower than that of plasma, water was added to the faecal sample.

5 The two stool charts were both recorded from patients on total 72-hour fasts. Chart A shows a progressive decline in stool weight, which is highly suggestive of an osmotic diarrhoea. Chart B shows only minor variations in the faecal weights with no significant decline from pre-fast levels, indicating secretory diarrhoea.

2a

3 Day Stool Weights: Fasting from Day 2				
Time	**Weight** (g)	**Consistency** Water, Custard Porridge, Toothpaste, Sausage	**Mucous** Lot Little None	**Blood** Lot Little None
DAY 1				
08:25	205	Custard	Nil	Nil
09:05	78	Porridge	Nil	Nil
09:30	156	Porridge	Nil	Nil
11:45	127	Porridge	Nil	Nil
17:50	283	Porridge	Nil	Nil
TOTAL	**849**			
DAY 2				
09:45	57	Porridge	Nil	Nil
12:00	189	Toothpaste	Nil	Nil
12:30	170	Toothpaste	Nil	Nil
14:30	95	Porridge	Nil	Nil
19:25	101	Porridge	Nil	Nil
TOTAL	**382**			
DAY 3				
9.45	88	Porridge	Nil	Nil
12.00	65	Toothpaste	Nil	Nil
14.30	115	Toothpaste	Nil	Nil
17.20	155	Toothpaste	Nil	Nil
TOTAL	**423**			

2b

3 Day Stool Weights: Fasting from Day 2				
Time	**Weight** (g)	**Consistency** Water, Custard Porridge, Toothpaste, Sausage	**Mucous** Lot Little None	**Blood** Lot Little None
DAY 1				
06:35	198	Water		
07:15	121	Water	Nil	Nil
0.8:55	319	Water	Nil	Nil
09:35	317	Water	Nil	Nil
11:30	106	Water	Nil	Nil
12:25	147	Water	Nil	Nil
15:15	213	Water	Nil	Nil
19:10	218	Water	Nil	Nil
TOTAL	**1639**			
DAY 2				
05:20	131	Water	Nil	Nil
09:15	173	Water	Nil	Nil
10:05	324	Water	Nil	Nil
10:30	243	Water	Nil	Nil
13:45	192	Water	Nil	Nil
19:00	98	Water	Nil	Nil
TOTAL	**1423**			
DAY 3				
07:45	123	Water	Nil	Nil
10:30	138	Water	Nil	Nil
12:50	78	Water	Nil	Nil
16:15	205	Water	Nil	Nil
18:30	200	Water	Nil	Nil
19:10	164	Water	Nil	Nil
20:30	144	Water	Nil	Nil
21:00	100	Water	Nil	Nil
22:10	94	Water	Nil	Nil
TOTAL	**1612**			

2a and **2b** Day stool weights: fasting from day 2.

3

	Na	K	Mg	Calculated Osmalality	Measured Osmolality	Osmolality Gap
A	105	36	6	282	296	14
B	96	44	48	280	378	102

3 Stool electrolytes and osmolality: Na = Sodium, K = Potassium, Mg = Magnesium — all at mmol/l.

4

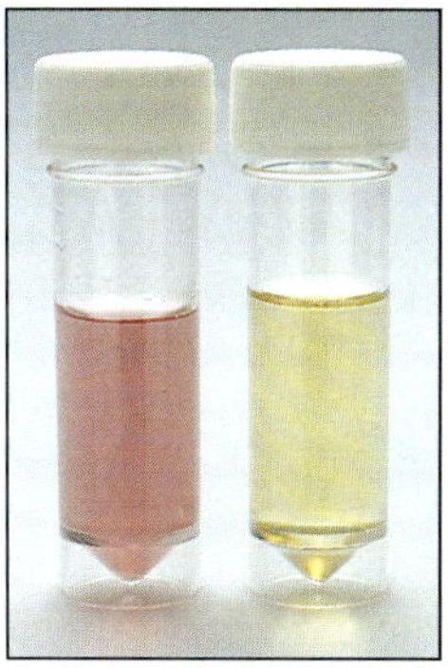

4 Urine test samples.

6 The common causes of an osmotic diarrhoea are lactose intolerance or other disaccharide deficiency, coeliac disease and osmotic laxative ingestion.
7 The two stool biochemical analyses are typical examples of both a secretory diarrhoea (**3**A) and an osmotic diarrhoea (**3**B). In chart A the product of twice the combined concentrations of the sodium and potassium ions is almost equal to the measured stool osmolality. Account is taken for chloride and bicarbonate ions by doubling the anion values. In chart B there is a large osmolar gap which is partly accounted for by the magnesium ion concentration. This patient had taken a magnesium-containing laxative.
8 The urine sample has been alkalinised by the addition of sodium hydroxide. The urine has turned a pinkish purple because it contained phenolpthalein(**4**). A similar colour change was seen when her faecal fluid was alkalinised. These findings suggest the patient has taken a laxative containing phenolpthalein.On direct confrontation the patient denied taking any laxative and was unwilling to have her bedside locker searched. She was unable to give any explanation for the findings and when asked if she wished to undergo further investigation, requested time alone to think about it. Shortly afterwards she was seen to leave the ward without any further comments to any member of the staff. On discussion with her parents it was learned that she had requested sweets and chocolate while she was on the 3-day fast. There was a problem between her and her fiancee but how this related to her laxative abuse was unclear. It is not uncommon for patients with laxative abuse to deny their ingestion. Many of the other non-osmotic laxatives can now be detected by screening urine by thin-layer chromatography.
9 There are many causes of a secretory diarrhoea. Many bacterial and viral infections stimulate intestinal secretion often by inducing adenyl-cyclase activity, usually by means of a toxin such as in Cholera. A variety of hormones which also act by this means such as VIP, Gastrin, Glucagon. Calcitonin and 5 Hydroxytryptamine induce intestinal secretion. Choloretic diarrhoea secondary to bile acid malabsorption by the terminal ileum, and some of the diarrhoea associated with bacterial overgrowth in the small intestine is also the result of induced intestinal secretion. A mechanism of diarrhoea in coeliac disease is also attributed to secretion, villous adenomas of the colon often secrete large amounts of mucus, and patients with inflammatory bowel disease also have a degree of secretory diarrhoea possibly related to prostaglandins.

Case 17

Constipation and a bad family history

This 54-year-old lady was referred from her general practitioner with a 6-week history of left iliac fossa discomfort, some abdominal bloating and a recent change in bowel habit with slight constipation. Normally she would open her bowels once per day without straining at stool. However, for the last 3 months she had only been opening them once in 2–3 days and had to strain. No bleeding nor passage of mucus was noted and she had not noticed any change in her appetite level, and had not lost any weight. The patient never smoked and drank alcohol within the accepted daily limits. Her family history was interesting (**1**). She was obviously very concerned about her change in bowel habit. On examination there was no significant abnormality found.

Investigations

Haematology and Biochemistry chart on page 73. Sigmoidoscopy (**2**).

1

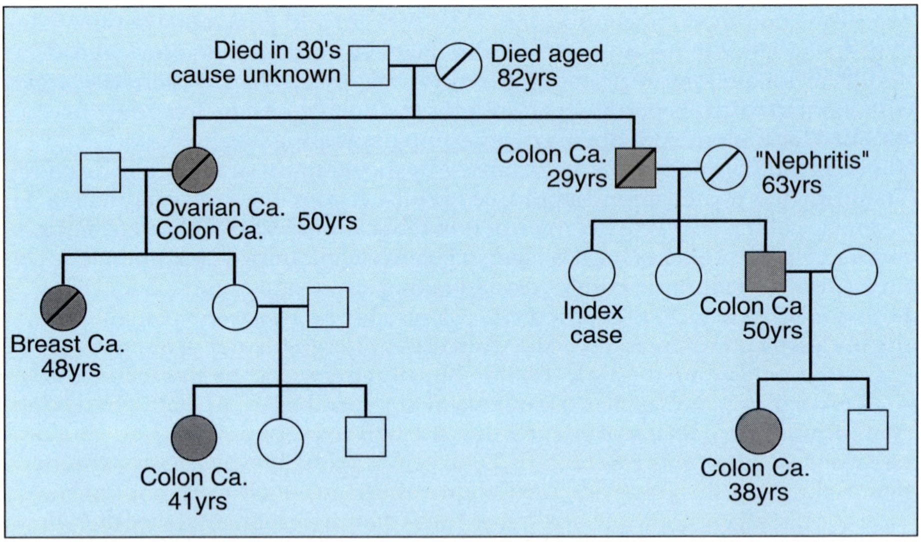

1 Patient's family history.

2

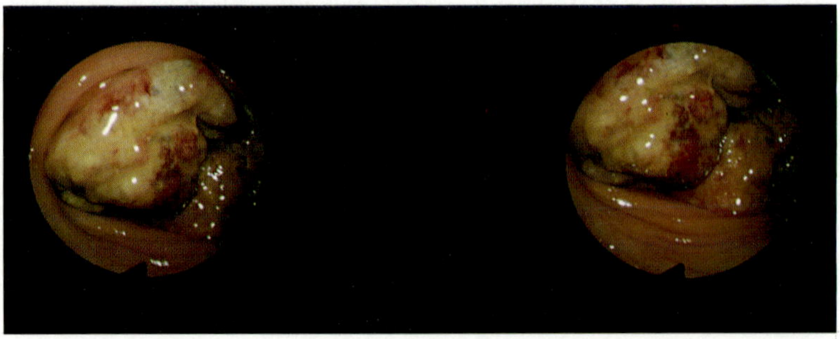

2 Sigmoidoscopy.

Questions

1 What does the family tree shown in **1** demonstrate about this family?
2 What does the sigmoidoscopy show?
3 What further investigations would you undertake ?
4 What inherited conditions might give rise to this sort of family history?
5 What treatment should be offered?

		Normal Range			Normal Range
Hb	10.2	11.5–16.0 **g/dl**	**MCHC**	29.2	33–36 **g/dl**
Hct	32.9	33–47 %	**Platelets**	353	150–400/ **10^9/l**
MCV	64.0	80–100 **fl**	**WCC**	9.2	3.5–11 **/ 10^9/l**
MCH	18.3	28–33 **pg**	**ESR**	22	< 20 **mm/hr**
Sodium	142	135–145 **mmol/l**	**Blood sugar**	5.8	3.5–7.2 **mmol/l**
Potassium	4.2	3.5–5.0 **mmol/l**	**Bilirubin**	4	2–17 **mmol/l**
Chloride	100	95–105 **mmol/l**	**Alk. Phos.**	122	35–125 **U/l**
Bicarbonate	25	20–30 **mmol/l**	**ALT**	25	0–35 **U/l**
Urea	3.9	2.5–7.0 **mmol/l**	**GGT**	45	0–35 **U/l**
Creatinine	93	50–150 **mmol/l**	**Albumin**	42	36–52 **g/l**
Phosphate	0.86	0.7–1.4 **mmol/l**	**Globulin**	30	22–32 **g/l**
Calcium	2.46	2.2–2.6 **mmol/l**	**CRP**	7	<5 **mg/l**

Answers and discussion

1 This patient is part of a family with a history of colon cancer in three generations. In addition several members of the family have had cancer in other organs, particularly gynaecological and breast cancer. The cancers are found in both males and females. It would thus appear that this patient is part of a family with a dominantly inherited tendency to bowel cancer, which is not sex linked.
2 The sigmoidoscopy shows a carcinoma of the colon which was found at 18 cm from the anal verge.
3 Investigation of this patient should be aimed at confirming the diagnosis, assessing the extent of spread, excluding other synchronous tumours and polyps in the colon and in advising her and her family about surveillance. In addition blood should be taken for genetic studies. Confirmation of the diagnosis is made by biopsying the tumour, and the histology is shown in **3**. Assessment of the extent of tumour spread is made by scanning the abdomen particularly to look for spread within the pelvis and to look for hepatic metastases. A chest x-ray should also be taken. Either ultrasound or CT scanning should be carried out preoperatively, and if dubious lesions are seen in the liver, magnetic resonance scans with or without Gadolinium enhancement may be of help.

Case 17

The next step before surgery should be examination of the whole colon to look for either synchronous polyps or tumours. This can either be accomplished by double-contrast barium-enema studies or by colonoscopy. The latter is the preferred method, because it allows biopsies to be taken and polyps to be endoscopically resected. Figure **4** demonstrates the technique of snare removal of an adenomatous polyp. In this patient the colonoscope could not be inserted higher than the tumour due to its stenosing effect on the bowel, and similarly a barium enema failed to outline the proximal colon due to the stricture, The patient had no evidence of hepatic, pulmonary or other spread .

4 The two most common syndromes with inherited colon cancer are familial adenomatous polyposis (FAP) previously known as Polyposis Coli, and Family Cancer Syndrome (Lynch Syndrome Type 1 or 2). The Lynch Syndrome Type 1 is inherited colon cancer within a family, whereas the Type 2 Syndrome includes families with gynaecological or breast cancer sufferers in the family. Peutz–Jehger Syndrome (**5**) of hamartomatous polyps is also associated with a slight risk of gastrointestinal cancer occurring in less than 5 % of cases. Inherited forms of colon cancer account for 5–10% of all colon cancers.

3

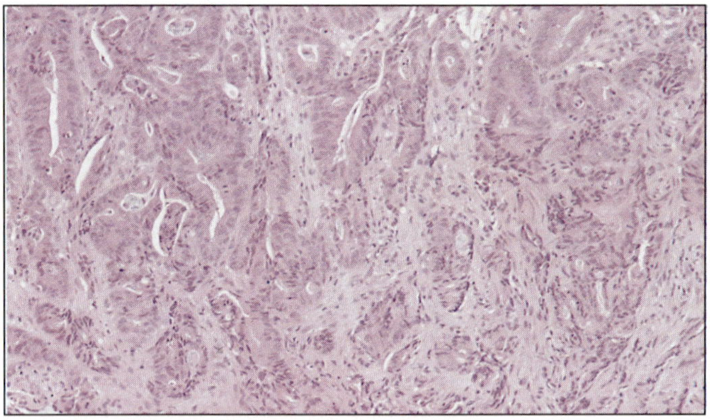

3 Histology of biopsy showing invasive adenocarcinoma.

4

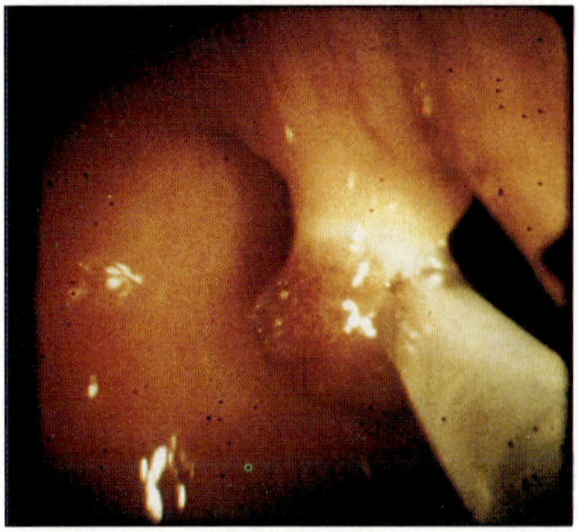

4 Snaring a colonic polyp.

5

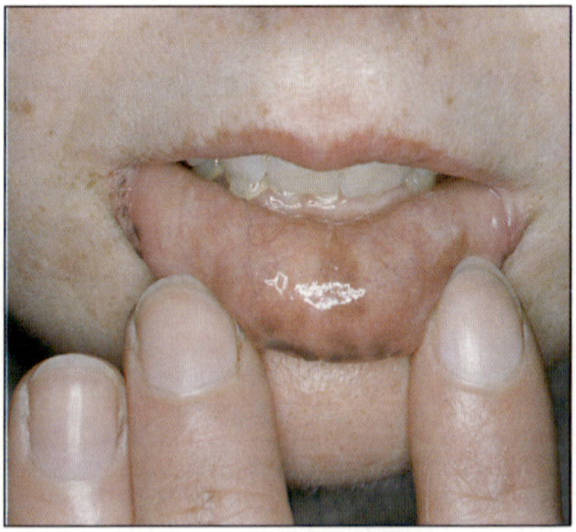

5 Mucocutaneous pigmentation in a patient with Peutz–Jehger syndrome.

5 The patient should be referred for surgery and should have a repeat colonoscopy shortly after the operation to ensure the remaining colon is clear. Thereafter, the patient should be enrolled on a long-term surveillance programme. This should be by means of regular annual or at the most biannual colonoscopy. Monitoring of blood CEA levels (Carcino–Embryonic-Antigen) is also of value, if elevated initially in looking for evidence of recurrence. Consideration should be given to adjuvant chemotherapy, because evidence is now increasingly showing this to be of value. The patient's sons should be counselled and screened for polyps or cancers and should be enrolled on a surveillance programme. Genetic markers may well show which members of a family are at risk.

The patient was thus referred for colonic resection at laparotomy. Laparotomy was performed and there was no evidence of spread outside the colon. An extended left hemicolectomy was carried out and the continuity of the bowel was restored by end-to-end anastomosis of the transverse colon to the upper rectum. There was no other lesion palpable in the remaining colon at operation. Histopathological examination of the resected colon revealed a tight stenosing carcinoma of the sigmoid, with an adjacent 1 cm diameter benign adenomatous polyp. Seven out of 10 resected lymph nodes were involved with carcinoma. The patient was offered and received outpatient chemotherapy as adjuvant treatment. A repeat colonoscopy at 3 months showed no polyps or cancers in the rest of the colon. One year later a repeat colonoscopy showed two polyps–one in the rectum just below the anastomosis and another in the proximal transverse colon. Snare polypectomy was performed and histology of one of these is shown below (**6**).

6

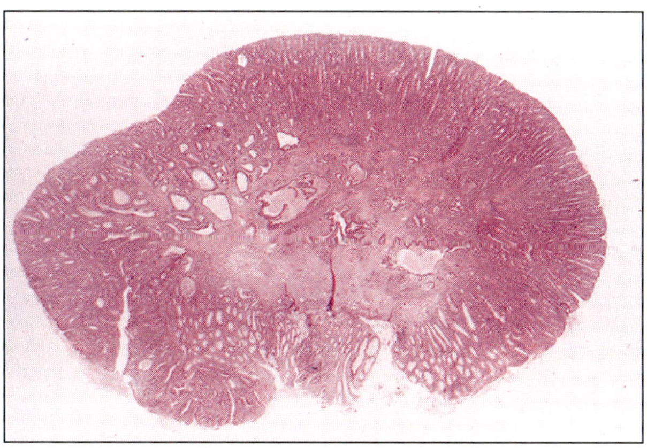

6 Histology of snare polypectomy.

Questions

6 What does the histology demonstrate ?
7 What would you advise with regards to treatment?

Answers and discussion

6 The histology shows an area of adenocarcinoma arising in a colonic polyp.
7 The patient should be offered further surgery to remove the cancers. If the cancers were confined to thc polyps and there was no evidence of invasion of the stalk, then snare polypectomy might be considered adequate in patients without a previous cancer or in patients with evidence of metastases. If there was no evidence of metastases, then consideration should be given to total colectomy and ileostomy, because the mucosa obviously has a 'field change' and there is a risk of the development of further cancers. This patient underwent total colectomy after detailed investigation to exclude metastases or lymph node involvement. At operation there was no evidence of recurrent cancer and none of the removed lymph nodes was involved. Three years later this patient was found at clinic attendance to have an elevated CEA level. Her liver scan (MRI) is shown (**7**).

Questions

8 What does the liver scan demonstrate?
9 How would you manage this patient?

7

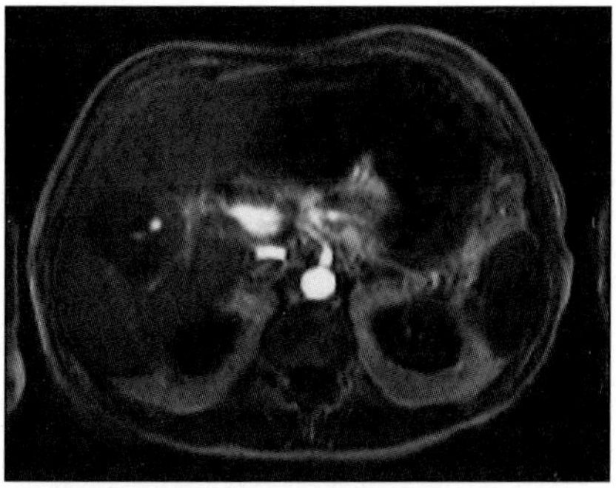

7 Liver scan of the patient.

Answers and discussion

8 There is a single low-density lesion in the right lobe of the liver consistent with a metastasis.
9 In a patient who develops a solitary metastasis from a colorectal primary, consideration must be given to resection which has been shown to prolong life. Indeed up to 3 metastases in a single lobe of the liver would not be a contra-indication. When such a lesion is seen, the patient is rescanned after 3 months and if no further deposits have appeared, then angiography is undertaken and if the patient is fit enough and there is no other evidence of spread, resection of the involved segments of liver undertaken by a surgeon specialising in this form of surgery. With modern equipment, such as ultrasonic dissectors and high-pressure water-jet dissectors partial hepatectomy can be accomplished with minimal blood loss and low mortality and morbidity. Other techniques are being developed for the management of single metastases such as interstitial laser therapy, cryo-probe treatment and alcohol injection.This patient had a partial hepatectomy and has had no further secondaries appear in the last 2 years.

Case 18

Dementia and jaundice

A 78-year-old patient was brought to the outpatient clinic from the nursing home where he had been living for 6 years. He had advanced Alzheimer's Disease, being dependent upon the nursing staff for feeding, washing and dressing. The nursing staff had noticed that he had not been eating as well as he did previously and that his urine had become darker and his stools paler. Just before his attendance at the clinic he had become more confused and had developed a pyrexia. It was thought that he had not had any pain. His past history was uninformative. On examination he was pyrexial with a temperature of 38·5°C and was jaundiced. There were no lymph nodes palpable and no signs of chronic liver disease. His abdomen was soft and non-tender and there were no masses palpable or organomegaly. There was a right subcostal scar presumed to be from a cholecystectomy. The scar was not recent.

Investigations

Haematology and Biochemistry chart on page 78. Straight x-ray of abdomen (**1**); Abdominal ultrasound (**2**).

1

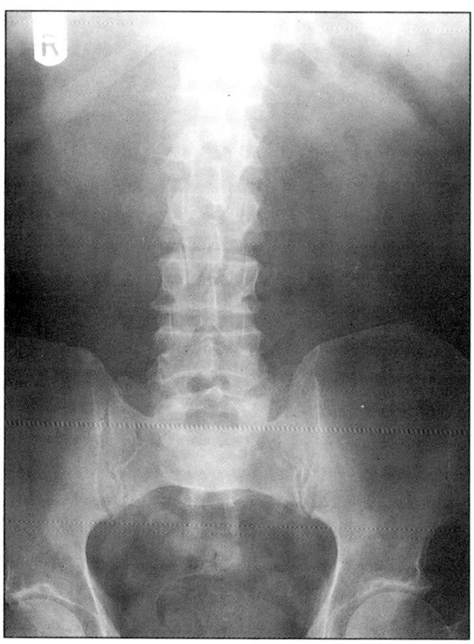

1 X-ray of abdomen.

2

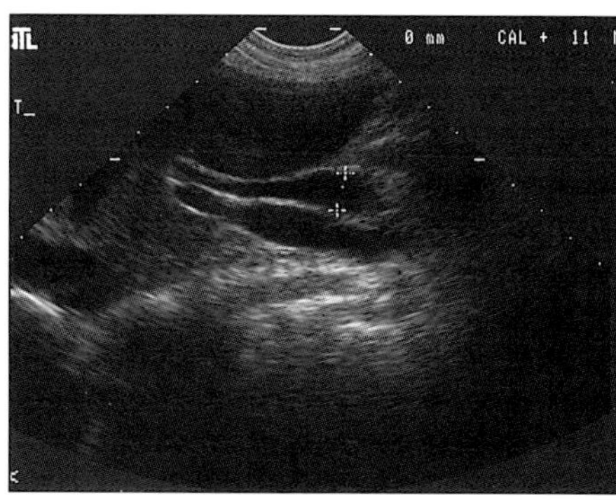

2 Ultrasound of the abdomen.

Questions

1 What are the likely diagnoses?
2 What other initial investigations are important?
3 What do the x-ray and ultrasound show?
4 What initial treatment would you give this patient?
5 What further investigations should be undertaken?

		Normal Range			Normal Range
Hb	11.9	12.5–18 **g/dl**	**MCHC**	34.7	33–36 **g/dl**
Hct	34.3	33–47 **%**	**Platelets**	322	150–400/ **10^9/l**
MCV	86.8	80–100 **fl**	**WCC**	14.7	3.5–11 **/ 10^9/l**
MCH	30.1	28–33 **pg**	**ESR**	58	< 20 **mm/hr**
Sodium	134	135–145 **mmol/l**	**Blood sugar**	6.3	3.5–7.2 **mmol/l**
Potassium	3.3	3.5–5.0 **mmol/l**	**Bilirubin**	179	2–17 **mmol/l**
Chloride	96	95–105 **mmol/l**	**Alk. Phos.**	635	35–125 **U/l**
Bicarbonate	22	20–30 **mmol/l**	**ALT**	104	0–35 **U/l**
Urea	3.8	2.5–7.0 **mmol/l**	**GGT**	890	0–35 **U/l**
Creatinine	52	50–150 **mmol/l**	**Albumin**	32	36–52 **g/l**
Phosphate	0.99	0.7–1.4 **mmol/l**	**Globulin**	36	22–32 **g/l**
Calcium	2.57	2.2–2.6 **mmol/l**	**CRP**	112	<5 **mg/l**

Answers and discussion

1 The two commonest causes of obstructive jaundice in a patient of this age are gallstones and carcinoma of the pancreas. In view of the fact that the patient has apparently had a cholecystectomy, it is probable that he has a retained common duct stone. The presence of a fever would favour the diagnosis of stone disease, because it is uncommon for patients with carcinoma of the pancreas, ampulla or bile ducts to have infected bile unless they have had some interventional technique performed with resultant induced infection. After such a long period it is unlikely that the jaundice is secondary to an operative problem such as suturing of a bile duct or a post operative stricture. In view of the fact that the patient lives in a nursing home it is important not to discount the possibility of a viral hepatitis.

2 In view of his pyrexia blood cultures should be taken as it is possible that he may have cholangitis. Serology for hepatitis A and B should be checked. A prothrombin time must be measured prior to any further more invasive investigation. A chest x-ray should be arranged to exclude a carcinoma of the bronchus.

3 The straight x-ray shows no evidence of a calculus in the region of the right upper quadrant however the ultrasound shows dilated extrahepatic ducts down to the level of the head of the pancreas. There is no acoustic shadow to suggest a stone in the lower common bile duct, nor is there any evidence of enlargement of the head of the pancreas or any other mass lesion.

4 The patient should be given intravenous fluids as it is unlikely that he would take enough orally. Evidence exists to suggest that renal failure secondary to obstructive jaundice is less likely if the patient is kept well hydrated. If the prothrombin time is prolonged, then the patient should be given an injection of vitamin K to prevent any haemorrhage at the time of any therapeutic procedure. In view of the pyrexia, in a patient with obstructive jaundice, it is wise to prescribe broad-spectrum antibiotics in case there is cholangitis.

The choice of antibiotics tends to change with time and availability of newer broader spectrum drugs. Amoxycillin, Metronidazole and Gentamicin were used widely, but more recently a combination of a third generation cephalosporin with gentamicin or ciprofloxacin alone has been used. It is important that the cover used extends to gram-negative organisms and that the antibiotic can enter bile. The final choice is often a matter of personal preference, but should probably be agreed with local microbiologists or infectious disease doctors. The most important decision is how next to investigate and treat the jaundice.

5 There are two main pathways of investigation and treatment in this case. Which one is chosen will depend upon the available facilities and the fitness of the patient.

The older route of investigation would be by means of a percutaneous thin needle cholangiogram to try to outline the biliary tract and define the aetiology of the obstruction. This route could be used for preoperative external biliary drainage by means of an indwelling catheter placed in situ at the time of the cholangiogram. If external biliary drainage is not undertaken at this time, the patient should be operated upon as soon as possible to relieve the biliary obstruction. The disadvantages of the use of fine needle cholangiography are the risk of introduction of infection and cholangitis, bleeding from the hepatic puncture sight and biliary leakage into the peritoneum with biliary peritonitis. Also, patient co-operation is helpful during this procedure.

Another more common approach is the use of Endoscopic Retrograde Cholangiography to both outline the cause of the obstruction and then to deal directly with it at the time of endoscopy. This approach is of particular relevance when avoidance of surgery is important as in the unfit patient. It is also ideally suited to patients who have obstruction secondary to stones where the gallbladder has been removed, and to the treatment of malignant biliary obstruction where resection is to be avoided or would be out of place. Figure **3** shows the result of the ERC in this patient. The adjacent figure (**4**) shows a typical percutaneous cholangiogram obtained in a similar patient.

Questions

6 What abnormality is seen in **3** and **4**?

7 What are the therapeutic options in treating this patient?

3

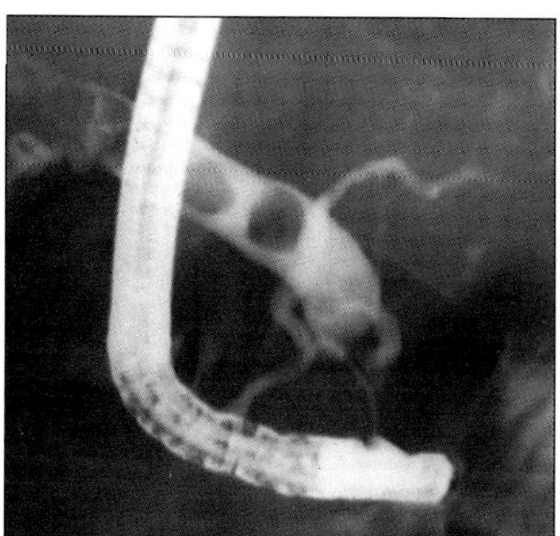

3 An ERC in progress.

4

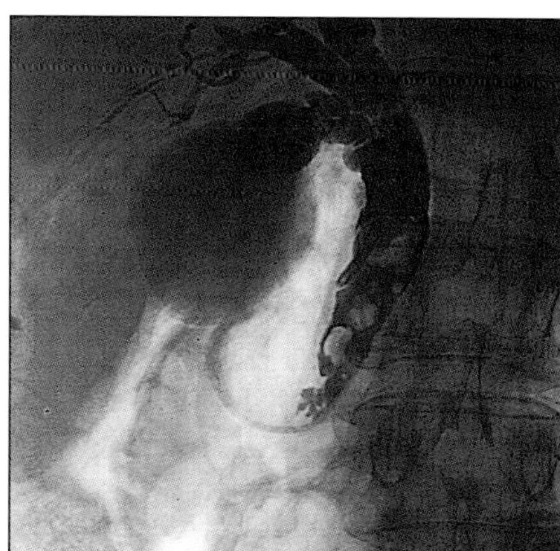

4 Cholangiogram.

Answers and discussion

6 Both x-rays show a dilated biliary tree with multiple gallstones within the common bile duct. Retained common duct stones is a common cause of extrahepatic biliary obstruction occurring usually late after cholecystectomy. Jaundice soon after cholecystectomy can be due to missed stones but may be caused by surgical damage to the bile duct or even hepatic ducts. There has been a recent spate of such cases with the introduction of laparoscopic cholecystectomy. Many surgeons now request preoperative ERCP before laparoscopic cholecystectomy, while others undertake peroperative cholangiography at laparoscopic cholecystectomy.

7 The therapeutic options in treating this patient are dependent upon the local facilities. At ERC in most units a sphincterotomy would be undertaken (**5**) and the stones removed by means of either a basket or by trawling the duct with a balloon (**6a–c**). Occasionally, the stones are either impacted or too large to be removed by these techniques. If this is the case, other techniques have to be

5

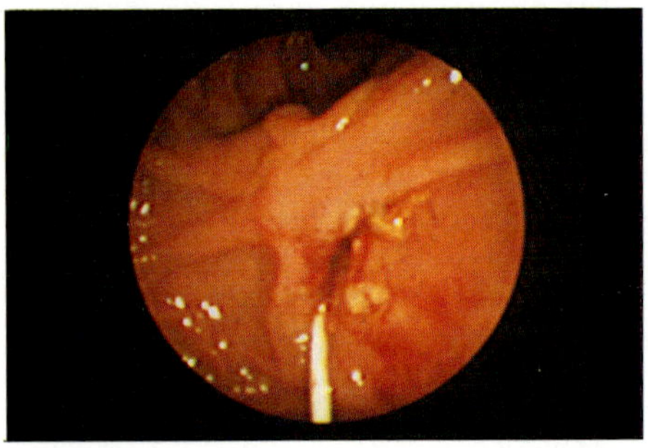

5 A sphincterotomy has been made and a balloon catheter is advanced into the duct to try and pull out any stones.

6a

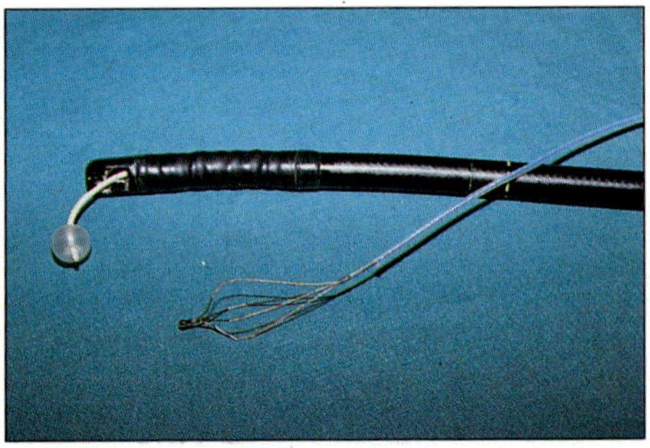

6 A balloon catheter and basket can be used to retrieve stones from the common bile duct.

6b

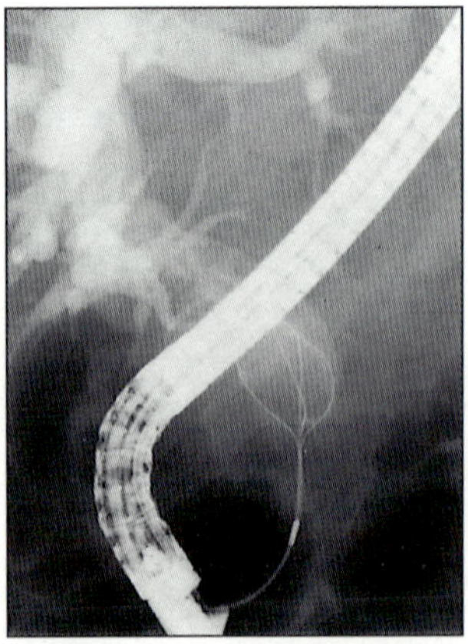

6b X-ray taken at ERC showing stone caught in a basket being withdrawn from common bile duct.

6c

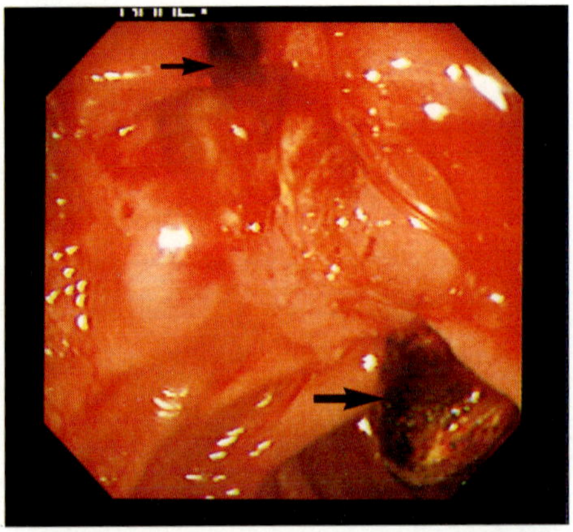

6c A sphincerotomy has been made (thin arrow) and a stone has been removed (thick arrow).

used. If ERC is not available and the diagnosis is made by percutaneous cholangiography, then as mentioned previously either early surgery or external drainage would be the options.

Question

8 What techniques can be used if stones in the common bile duct are impacted or too large to be removed via the sphincterotomy?

Answer and discussion

8 The most common technique is to try and crush the stones with a mechanical lithotripter. This is a strong wire basket in a flexible wire sheath (**7**). When the stone is caught in the basket the ratchet handle is wound up, withdrawing the basket towards the sheath tip, crushing the stone. This is effective but there are technical problems with the snare which sometimes prevents success. Another option is to use a mother and baby scope (**8**) and under direct visualisation either attempt to disrupt or crack the stone by an electro-hydraulic lithotripter or by use of a pulsed YAG or Alexandrite laser.

7

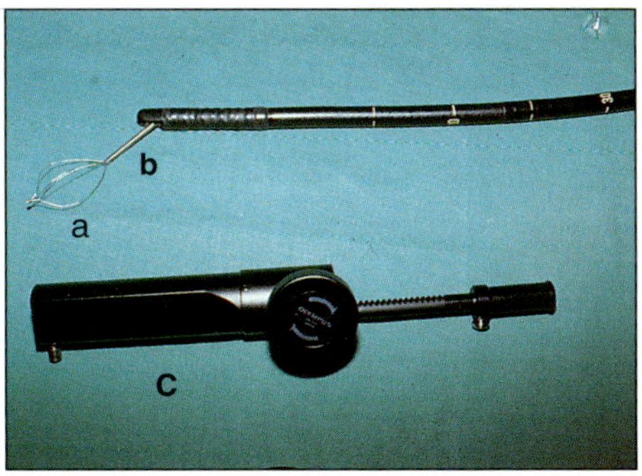

7 Lithrotripsy basket. (**a**) Wire basket. (**b**) Metal sheath against which the basket closed, so crushing the stone. (**c**) The device used to put traction on the wire basket.

8

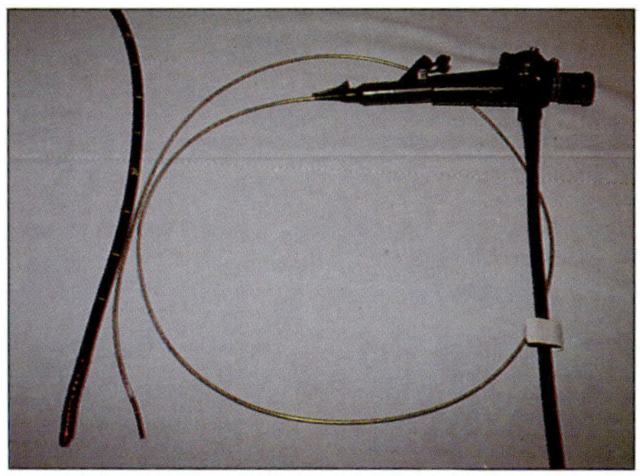

8 A 'baby' enteroscopic choledochoscope which can be passed down the biopsy channel of the duodenoscope (shown on left).

If these methods are unavailable or do not work, or if surgery is to be avoided, the choice lies between placing a pigtailed stent around the stone to prevent it impacting and blocking the bile duct or placing a nasobiliary drain in above the stone (**9** and **10**). If the pigtail stent is used, then this is left in situ and is changed only if the jaundice returns or there are further episodes of cholangitis. The nasobiliary drain is used to temporarily drain the biliary tract and can be used to try and flush small stones out into the duodenum; or for larger stones it can be used to try and dissolve them by using a solvent such as mono-octanoin. Yet another use of a nasobiliary drain is to permit easy cholangiographic localisation of the gallstones to enable Extra-Corporeal Shock-Wave Lithotripsy to be undertaken, if as in this case the gallstone was ultrasonically invisible (**11**).This patient had his stones removed by use of a basket and balloon after a sphincterotomy and his health improved rapidly.

9

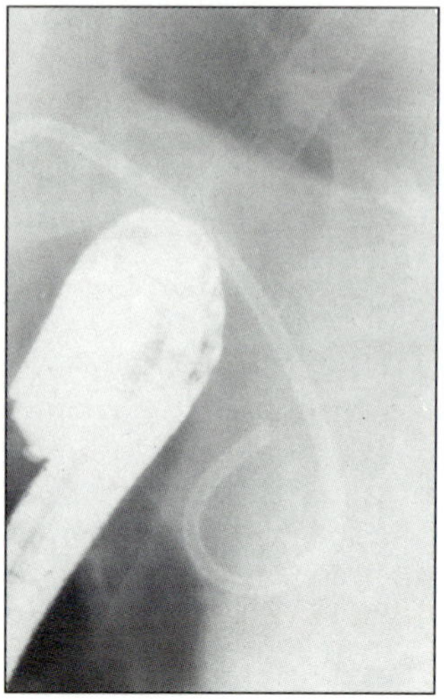

10

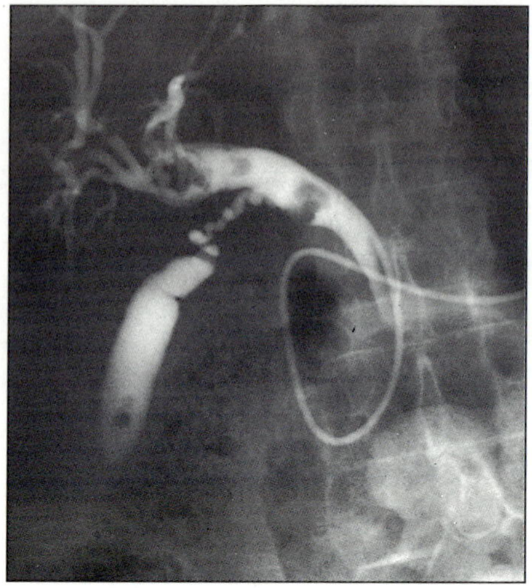

9 Pigtail stent placed in common bile duct.

10 Nasobiliary drain.

11

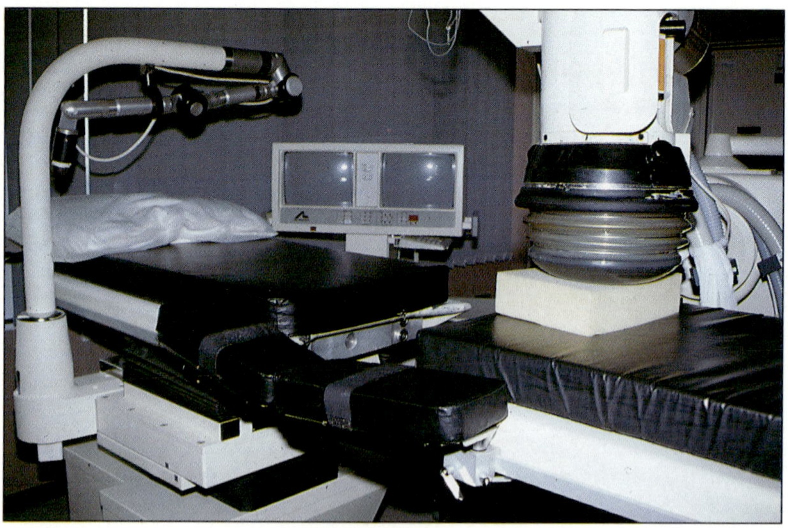

11 Extracorporeal shock wave lithotriptor.

Case 19

Weight loss and jaundice

A 58-year-old man presented with central upper abdominal pain and anorexia of 5 weeks duration. He had lost a few pounds in weight but felt quite fit otherwise. The pain seemed to come on after food initially but gradually had become more persistent. He denied any heartburn or dysphagia and had no other symptoms of note. He used to drink up to 50 units of alcohol per week but had reduced this some months before on the advice of a friend. The patient had been a smoker for 40 years and was using 20–30 cigarettes per day. On examination there was no significant abnormality and in particular no mass or abdominal tenderness.

Questions

1 His primary care physician had given him a trial of an H_2 blocker without success, was this reasonable?
2 What initial investigations would you undertake?

Answers and discussion

1 Although the counsel of perfection would be for every patient to have a definitive diagnosis made before the start of therapy, in most countries this is not practical. Therefore, it is reasonable to give a patient a short trial of a relevant treatment if the diagnosis appears clear. In this patient the history was atypical. Whenever a trial of blind treatment is being undertaken, it is important for the doctor to exclude those patients with sinister symptoms such as weight loss, dysphagia, bleeding or anaemia. On these grounds this patient should have been investigated first. Finally, patients presenting with dyspepsia for the first time over 40 years of age should be considered for investigation to ensure that the patient does not have an underlying malignancy. In some countries potent drugs can only be prescribed after a definitive diagnosis has been established.
2 Initial investigation should include a full blood count, chest x-ray and probably basic biochemical investigations, such as liver function tests in view of his previous heavy alcohol intake. A gastroscopy or double-contrast barium meal would be appropriate.

Investigations

Haematology and Biochemistry chart on page 84; Chest x-ray (**1**); Oesophago-gastro-duodenoscopy: view of antrum and pylorus(**2**).

1

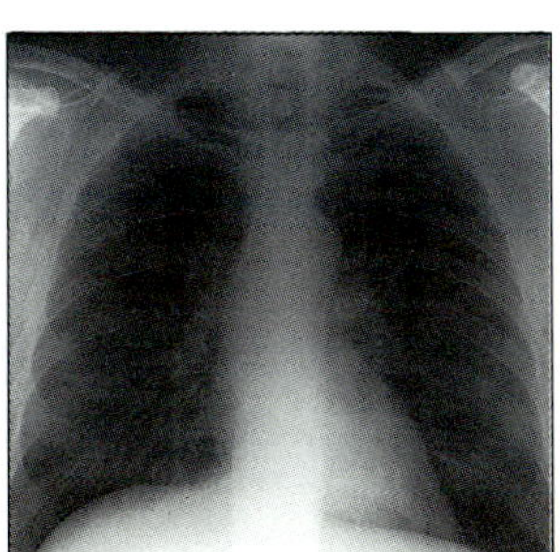

1 Chest x-ray.

2

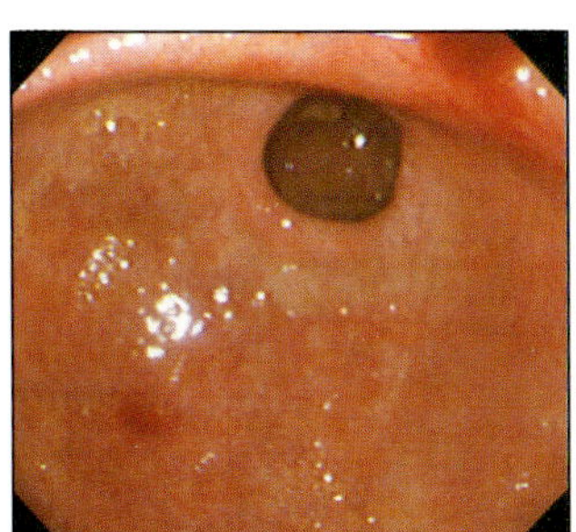

2 Duodenoscopy.

Case 19

		Normal Range			Normal Range
Hb	13.0	12.5–18 **g/dl**	**MCHC**	33.5	33–36 **g/dl**
Hct	38.9	33–47 **%**	**Platelets**	358	150–400/ **10^9/l**
MCV	36.9	80–100 **fl**	**WCC**	8.1	3.5–11 **/ 10^9/l**
MCH	29.1	28–33 **pg**	**ESR**	10	< 20 **mm/hr**
Sodium	142	135–145 **mmol/l**	**Blood sugar**	5.5	3.5–7.2 **mmol/l**
Potassium	4.4	3.5–5.0 **mmol/l**	**Bilirubin**	16	2–17 **mmol/l**
Chloride	105	95–105 **mmol/l**	**Alk. Phos.**	142	35–125 **U/l**
Bicarbonate	26	20–30 **mmol/l**	**ALT**	28	0–35 **U/l**
Urea	4.4	2.5–7.0 **mmol/l**	**GGT**	24	0–35 **U/l**
Creatinine	93	50–150 **mmol/l**	**Albumin**	38	36–52 **g/l**
Phosphate	1.05	0.7–1.4 **mmol/l**	**Globulin**	32	22–32 **g/l**
Calcium	2.30	2.2–2.6 **mmol/l**	**CRP**	<5	<5 **mg/l**

Questions

3 Does the chest x-ray show any abnormality?
4 What does the endoscopy show?
5 What further investigations would you undertake in this patient?

Answers and discussion

3 The chest x-ray is normal.

4 The gastroscopy shows mild antral hyperaemia which is patchy and consistent with mild gastritis. Although it is possible that this might account for his symptoms, such endoscopic changes are common and persistent pain and weight loss would not usually be caused by gastritis of this degree. The endoscopic assessment of the severity of gastritis is difficult and particularly in mild disease is very subjective. Histology can be of help in ascertaining the degree of inflammation.

5 This patient has thus got a mildly raised alkaline phosphatase with persistent abdominal pain and mild weight loss, The endoscopy has not revealed the likely cause and further investigation is indicated. An ultrasound examination of the upper abdomen would be appropriate, and in many countries this is undertaken as a bedside procedure by the gastroenterologist when the patient is first seen. Figure **3** shows his scan.

Questions

6 What does the scan demonstrate?
7 What investigations would you undertake next?

Answers and discussion

6 The scan shows mildly dilated intrahepatic bile ducts. There was gas obscuring the pancreas and the lower end of the bile duct was not visualised. No gall stones were seen in the gall bladder.

3 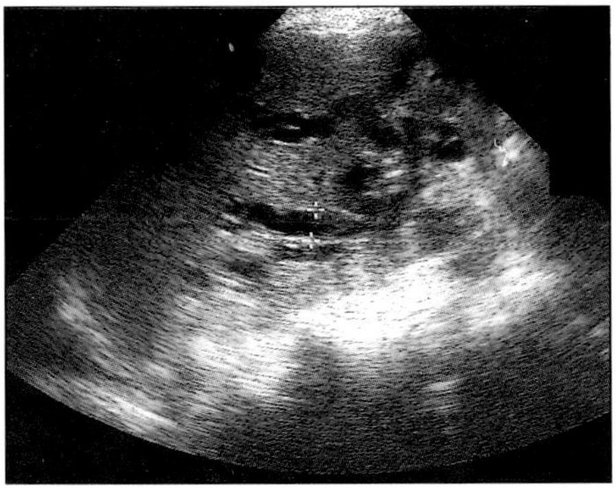

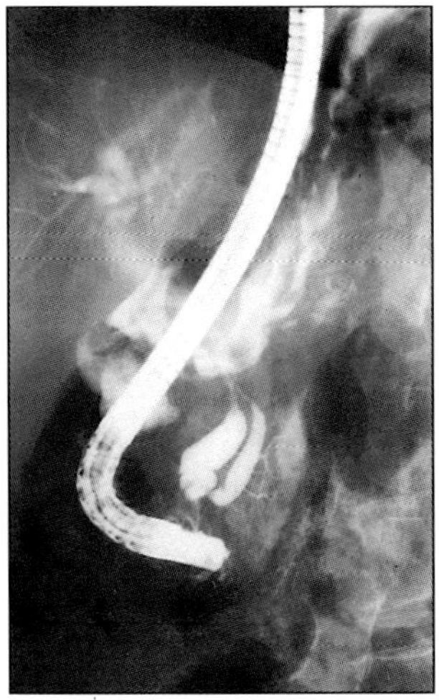 4

3 Ultrasound scan of liver.

4 Result of the patient's ERCP.

7 Repeat liver function tests would be reasonable to assess if there is rapid obstruction of the biliary tract, as well as measurement of the prothrombin time. The next most essential investigation is to outline the cause of the biliary obstruction.The method most often chosen is by ERCP; however, if the facilities do not exist for this procedure, percutaneous transhepatic cholangiography is a another method, but suffers from the risks of bleeding or bile leak from the puncture site. In addition, unless the radiologist is highly skilled, therapy by this route is more difficult and where such skill does not exist, the patient might need to be referred straight for surgery.This patient underwent ERCP and the result is shown in **4**.

Questions

8 What does the ERCP x-ray film demonstrate?
9 How would you manage this patient in view of these findings?

Answers and discussion

8 The x-ray demonstrates the classical double duct sign, with occlusion of both the common bile duct and the pancreatic duct . This finding strongly suggests a tumour in the head of the pancreas but could be due to a cyst or other mass lesion.

9 There are two parts to the management of this patient. The first aim is to relieve the biliary obstruction, to prevent the jaundice deepening (The second set of investigations show the bilirubin to have risen with a deterioration in the alkaline phoshatase and other enzymes). The second aim is to confirm the diagnosis of the obstructing lesion and assess whether the lesion is resectable. In most centres at the time of the ERCP when an obstructed biliary tract is discovered attempts would be made to overcome the obstruction. This patient had several prolonged attempts made to get a guide wire through the obstruction with a view to placing a stent through the obstruction endoscopically. Despite an adequate sphincterotomy and the use of several different forms of guide wire, all attempts failed. It was decided that as the degree of jaundice was not great, no further drainage procedures should be undertaken until the cause and extent of the obstructing lesion was confirmed. The most likely cause for the obstructed

biliary and pancreatic ducts is a carcinoma of the head of the pancreas. It is essential to assess both the size and to look for evidence of spread before embarking on surgical exploration. As an ultrasound scan had been obscured by overlying bowel gas, either a CT scan or perhaps an MR scan would be the next step. Figure **5** shows the CT scan in this patient. If the lesion is small, and there are no signs of local or distant spread, then consideration should be given to surgery. Many pancreatic surgeons will request angiography as a prelude to ensure that there is no vascular encroachment or invasion that would preclude surgery. The angiogram is also of value as a 'route map' at the time of surgery, and to demonstrate any aberrations of vascular supply. The use of pancreatic tumour markers such as CA 19–9 or CAM 17.1 is of value if there is debate about the nature of the lesion, and in some centres percutaneous fine-needle aspiration biopsy of mass lesions either at ERCP, using the obstructed ducts as an aiming guide or at scanning is the routine.This patient went on to arteriography, a selected film of which is shown in **6**.

Questions

10 What does the CT scan show?
11 What does the arteriogram demonstrate?

5

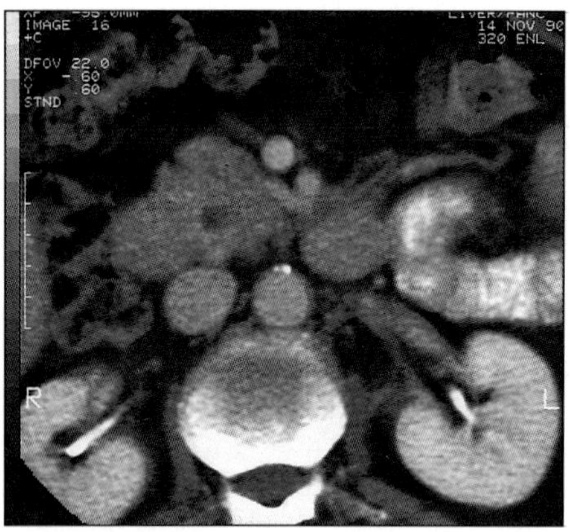

5 CT scan.

6

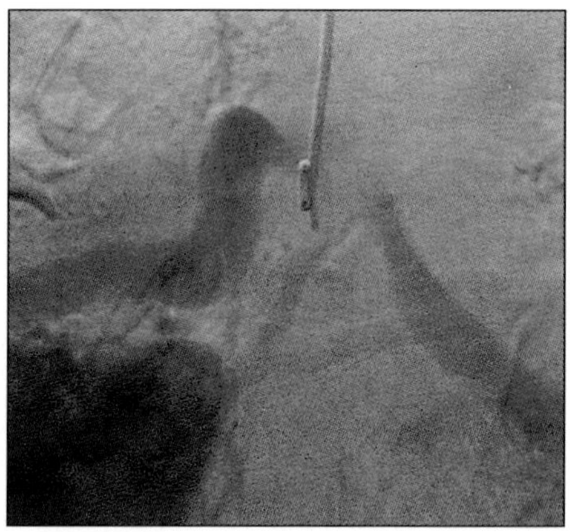

6 Arteriogram.

Answers and discussion

10 The CT scan shows a mass lesion of mixed density in the head of the pancreas. There was no evidence of lymphadenopathy.
11 The angiogram shows encroachment of the tumour on the coeliac axis and superior mesenteric vein. These findings are taken to signify that the tumour is inoperable.

Question

12 How would you proceed at this point?

Answer and discussion

12 The patient clearly needs palliative care both to relieve his pain and the increasing jaundice. Pain relief is very important and adequate doses of analgesia

upto and including opiates may be necessary. If such simple therapy fails, then the addition of non-steroidal anti-inflammatory drugs can be of benefit. Local nerve blocks such as coeliac plexus block with alcohol may be of help but needs to be performed by an expert in this field, usually a member of a dedicated pain-relief service. Relief of the jaundice can be achieved in three ways. The first would be a repeat attempt at ERC in the hope of being more successful in traversing the stricture. The second is to attempt to bypass the stricture from above at percutaneous cholangiography, and the third is to arrange for surgical bypass. It was decided in this patient to proceed to percutaneous cholangiography. A guide wire was manipulated through the dilated duct system and was passed into the duodenum (**7**). It was decided that instead of passing a stent down through the liver from above an ERC/Combined procedure should be undertaken. The protruding guide wire in the duodenum was picked up in a snare and withdrawn up through the mouth. Over the guide wire a stenting side-viewing duodenoscope was passed and a stent inserted through the stricture to relieve the obstruction (**8**). If such a combined procedure was not available and the radiologist had the necessary skills, then after suitable dilatation over the guide wire, a stent might have been inserted percutaneously through the liver. This is a slightly more uncomfortable procedure for the patient and has a greater morbidity. Had the guide wire not been placed through the obstruction, either external drainage could be used preoperatively or a further attempt made at placing the guide wire after drainage and decompression of the bile ducts. It is not uncommon for a second attempt to be successful, possibly because of relief of oedema or due to slight changes in orientation of the bile duct with relief of the distension. Surgery is indicated if there is any degree of duodenal obstruction in addition to the bile duct obstruction, if there is doubt about the diagnosis or about resectability. In centres without interventional radiology or endoscopy, then surgical drainage is the mainstay. This patient had a successful combined approach and a stent was placed through the stricture with complete relief of the obstruction. At present there is no good evidence that either radiotherapy or chemotherapy has a place in the treatment of carcinoma of the pancreas, but new combinations of drugs with or without radiotherapy are being tried.

7

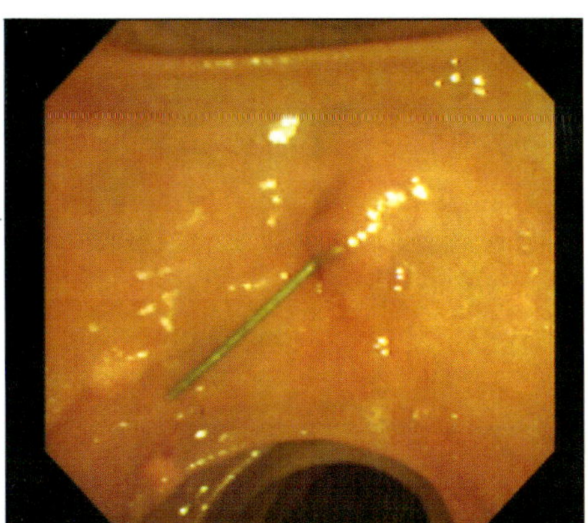

7 Wire protruding through ampulla after percutaneous placement.

8

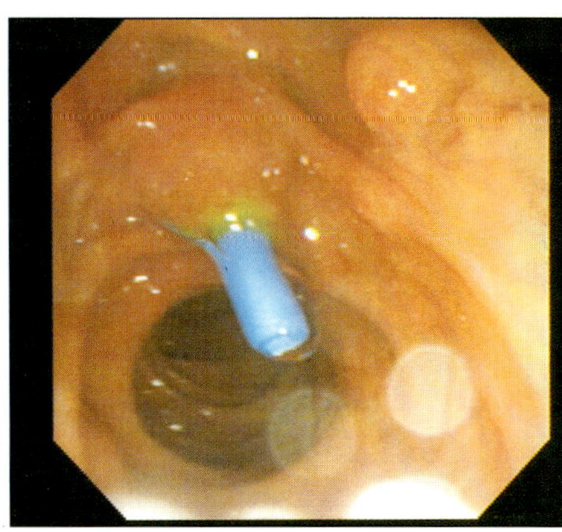

8 Positon of stent after endoscopic placement.

Case 20

Bloody diarrhoea and bone pain

A 68-year-old lady was admitted to the hospital with an 8-week history of progressively increasing diarrhoea. At the start the diarrhoea did not contain any blood, but within a week of admission blood and mucus was present in every motion. She had colicky lower abdominal pain made worse by, and after defaecation, and had developed tenesmus. She had felt increasingly weak for the fortnight before admission and had considerable difficulty walking, going up stairs and getting out of a chair. Her appetite had been poor for the 8 weeks and she had lost over 5 kg. For the preceding few months she had complained of mouth ulcers and just before admission had developed a painless ulcerated area on her thigh (**1**). On examination she looked unwell, and had a diffusely tender abdomen without guarding.

Investigations

Haematology and Biochemistry chart on page 89. Sigmoidoscopy to 20 cm (**2**).

1

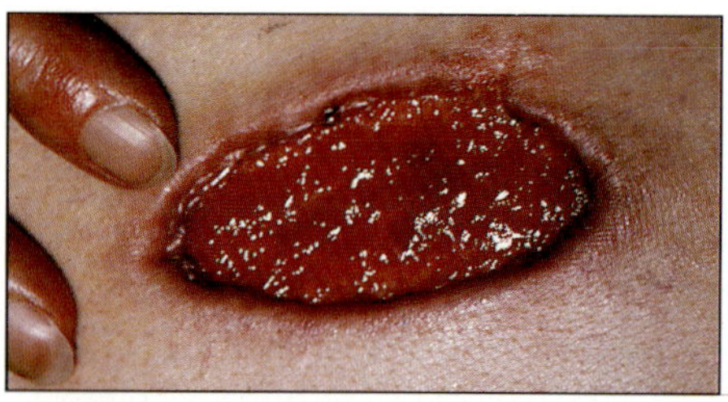

1 Painless ulceration on the thigh.

2

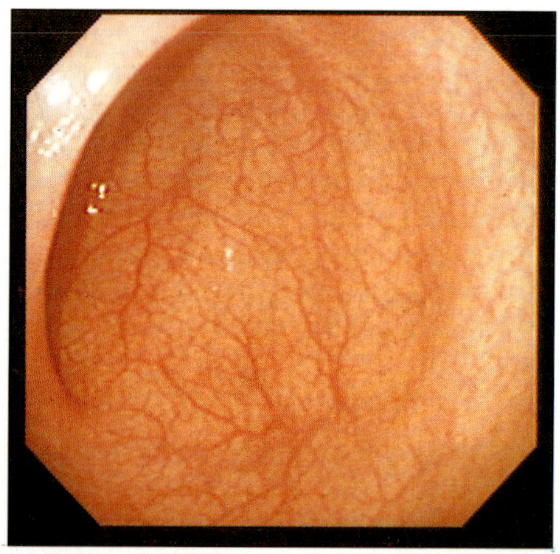

2 Sigmoidoscopy.

3

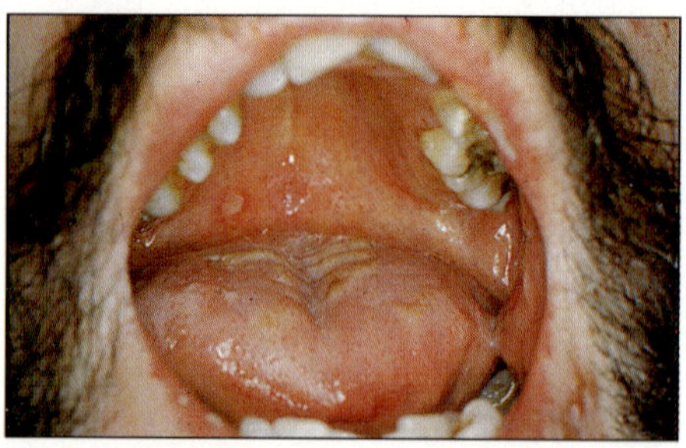

3 Apthous ulceration in a different patient with inflammatory bowel disease.

Questions

1 What is the differential diagnosis ?

2 What is the skin lesion and what are the other cutaneous manifestations of the likely diagnosis ?

3 What does the sigmoidoscopy show and does this affect your diagnosis, and if so how ?

4 What further investigations would you undertake ?

5 What initial treatment would you give ?

		Normal Range			Normal Range
Hb	11.2	11.5–16.0 **g/dl**	**MCHC**	33.4	33–36 **g/dl**
Hct	32	33–47 **%**	**Platelets**	454	150–400/ **10^9/l**
MCV	75.8	80–100 **fl**	**WCC**	4.4	3.5–11 **/ 10^9/l**
MCH	25.3	28–33 **pg**	**ESR**	57	< 20 **mm/hr**
Sodium	141	135–145 **mmol/l**	**Blood sugar**	3.8	3.5–7.2 **mmol/l**
Potassium	2.6	3.5–5.0 **mmol/l**	**Bilirubin**	8	2–17 **mmol/l**
Chloride	107	95–105 **mmol/l**	**Alk. Phos.**	159	35–125 **U/l**
Bicarbonate	30	20–30 **mmol/l**	**ALT**	9	0–35 **U/l**
Urea	6.3	2.5–7.0 **mmol/l**	**GGT**	18	0–35 **U/l**
Creatinine	71	50–150 **mmol/l**	**Albumin**	29	36–52 **g/l**
Phosphate	0.56	0.7–1.4 **mmol/l**	**Globulin**	24	22–32 **g/l**
Calcium	2.24	2.2–2.6 **mmol/l**	**CRP**	124	<5 **mg/l**

Answers and discussion

1 The differential diagnosis based on the history must include both idiopathic inflammatory bowel disease (ulcerative colitis or Crohn's), infective colitides, a carcinoma or large villous adenoma. Ischaemic colitis is another possibility. The history of apthoid ulcers (**3**) (NB: a different patient), and the skin lesion would favour a diagnosis of inflammatory bowel disease.

2 The skin lesion shown in **1** is pyoderma gangrenosum. This is commonly associated with inflammatory bowel disease, either ulcerative colitis or Crohn's. Other skin lesions seen with these conditions are erythema nodosum (**4**) and occasionally a vasculitic rash. Psoriasis is found with an increased incidence in Crohn's disease.

3 The sigmoidoscopy was entirely normal, apart from the presence of diarrhoea. The vascular pattern was preserved and biopsy was normal. The presence of rectal sparing should suggest either a focal colitis such as Crohn's colitis or an ischaemic colitis occurring higher up the colon. A neoplasm occurring higher up would also have a normal sigmoidoscopy.

4 It is important to exclude an infective cause for the bloody diarrhoea and thus stool samples should be sent urgently for microbiological study. This should include specific requests to exclude *Campylobacter, Yersinia, Clostridium difficile, Salmonella, Shigella* and *Amoebae.* The next most important investigation is to look for evidence of ulceration and inflammation in the rest of the colon, as well as excluding an adenoma or cancer. Either an instant barium enema, or colonoscopy should be performed. Both of these need to be carried out with care in a patient with acute colitis, the colonoscopy does however allow biopsies to be taken. Figure **5** shows the barium enema.

5 Initial treatment should be aimed at restoring the patients electrolytes to normality with either oral potassium supplements, or if the patient is nauseated

or unable to tolerate the oral therapy, with intravenous potassium. In patients with more profound anaemia transfusion should be undertaken.

Once infection has been excluded, and colitis, be that ulcerative colitis or Crohn's colitis, has been confirmed, it is reasonable to start more specific therapy. This will usually be by use of steroids and sulphasalazine or one of the newer 5-aminosalicylic acid derivatives. Limited proctocolitis may respond simply to rectal steroids in the form of either a foam or enema. More extensive colitis usually requires oral steroids, whilst for those patients who are acutely ill intravenous steroids are most often used. Sulphasalazine or the newer derivatives without the sulphonamide moiety also can be used for the

4

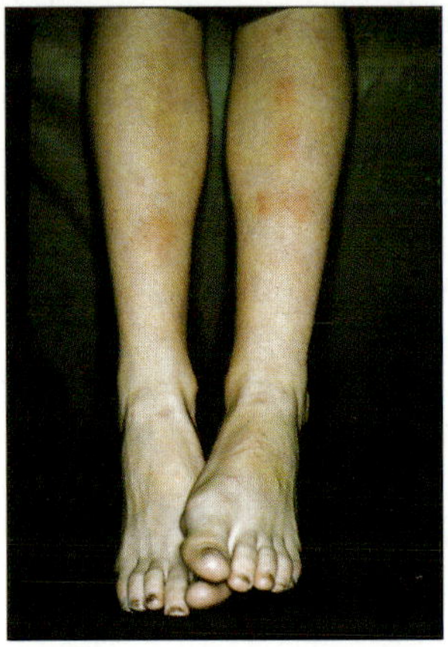

4 Erythema nodosa.

5

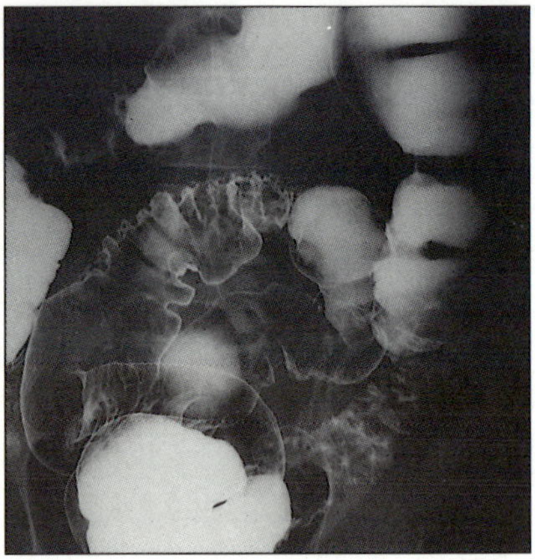

5 Barium enema.

treatment of an acute attack, although more usually people think of them as drugs used for maintenance and prevention of relapse. Considerable interest has been shown in the dietary management of colitis and Crohn's colitis. There is no absolute agreement. However, many gastroenterologists use liquid enteral feeds either alone or with the more conventional drug treatments referred to above in the treatment of an acute attack of idiopathic inflammatory bowel disease. For ulcerative colitis there is less evidence that this form of therapy works, but for Crohn's colitis it is more a matter of debate as to which diet rather than whether a diet should be used. There are probably slightly more papers in favour of the use of a true elemental diet than for a protein hydrolysate based diet in acute Crohn's. In those patients with fulminant disease parenteral nutrition is the most appropriate form of nutrition as well as offering 'complete bowel rest'.

Questions

6 What does the barium enema show?
7 What are the local complications of Crohn's disease?
8 Figures **6** and **7** are examples of complicated Crohn's disease. What do they demonstrate?

Answers and discussion

6 The barium enema shows the typical appearances of Crohn's disease affecting the colon. There are skip lesions and areas of deep ulceration.
7 The local complications of Crohn's disease are the formation of fistulae,

stricturing and abscess formation. Bleeding can occur but is rarely torrential, and spontaneous perforation can also occur rarely.

8 Figure **6** shows a vesico-colic fistula in a young woman with Crohn's colitis. Figure **7** shows a complex of fistulae centred around the terminal ileum of a patient with long-standing terminal ileal Crohn's disease.

6
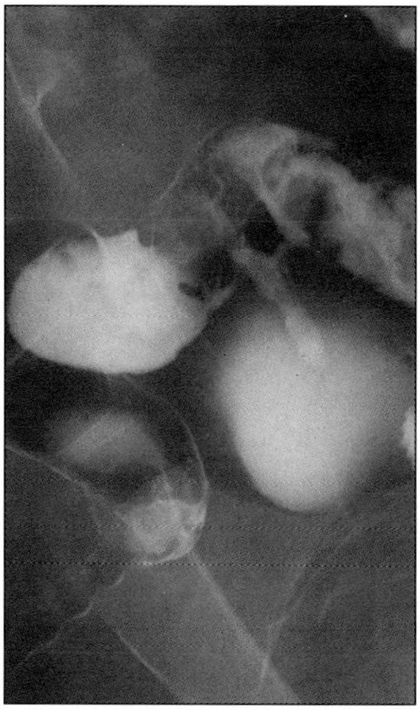

6 A vesico-colic fistula.

7
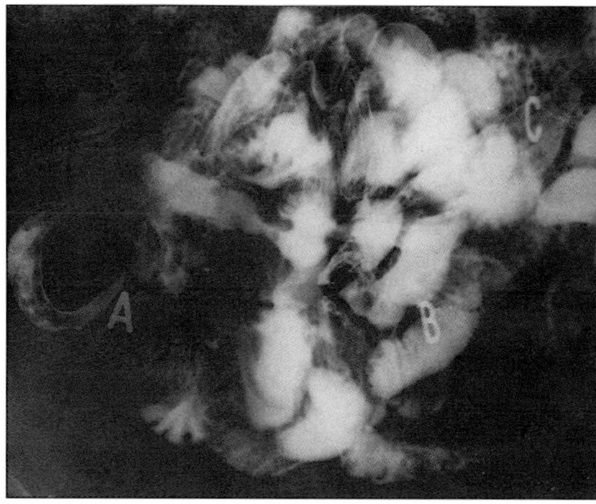

7 Complex fistulae and strictures in longstanding Crohn's disease. A–C are exit points of entrocutaneous fistulae.

Progress

The patient settled rapidly on intravenous steroids and elemental feeding and was discharged 2 weeks later. Sulphasalazine and steroids were prescribed. Over the next 8 years she had several relapses and was rarely off steroids for more than a few months. She then presented again with a further attack of pain and diarrhoea. Further investigation was carried out (**8**). At this admission she also complained of severe pain in the left groin and hip area, so much so that walking was difficult. An x-ray of her pelvis is shown in **9**.

Questions

9 What is the investigation shown in **8**, and why is it used?
10 What does the pelvic x-ray show and what are the possible causes?
11 What other causes of pain in the hip might this patient have?

Answers and discussion

9 The investigation shows a radionucleide scan with uptake of the isotope in the liver, spleen and most of the descending colon. This is a labelled white-cell study used to delineate the extent of inflammation in both the small and large bowel, as well as for looking for abscesses. The patient's own white cells are incubated with $Indium^{111}$ or $Technetium^{99}$ and are re-injected into the patient. The patient is scanned at 3 and 24 hours and persistence of the isotope suggests inflammation in the bowel wall or abscess formation. The

8 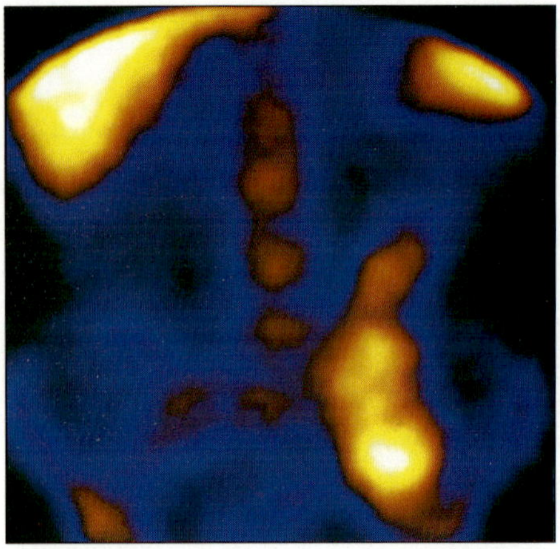

8 A scan.

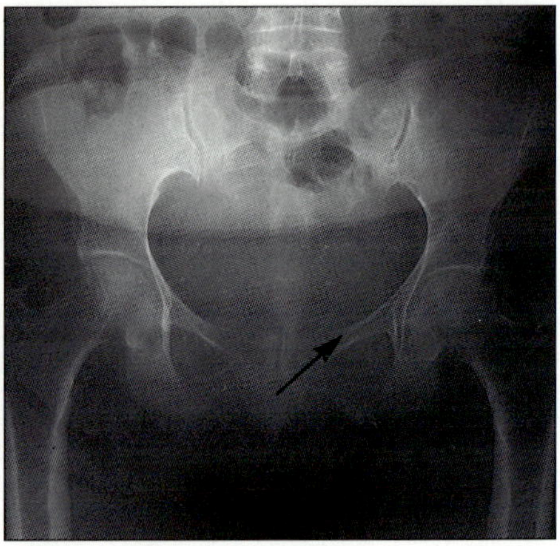 9

9 X-ray of the pelvic region.

investigation is less upsetting to a patient than a barium contrast study, particularly if the perineal region is tender due to abscesses or fistulae, or if they are unable to tolerate small-bowel intubation or swallow oral barium for a small-bowel study. The investigation gives an overall assessment of the inflamed areas but unlike with barium studies, does not give precise structural detail.

10 The x-ray shows a fracture in the pubic ramus (arrow). The possibilities are that this is traumatic, perhaps as a result of osteoporosis from the steroids, although there was no history of trauma, that it is the site of a pathological fracture through a metastatic deposit, or that it is a pseudo fracture (Looser zone). This patient was investigated fully and no underlying malignancy was found, and on CT scanning it was thought that the area of abnormality was a Looser zone. The patient was found to have low vitamin D levels and a raised alkaline phosphatase of bony origin. It was assumed that her osteomalacia was due to malabsorption but detailed small-bowel studies failed to confirm the presence of Crohn's disease macroscopically in the small bowel on either labelled white-cell scanning or on small-bowel radiology. Jejunal biopsies were also normal. The patient was of Indian descent, having lived in the UK for 30 years. She originated from Gudjurat and had kept to a traditional diet. It was proposed that the lack of sunshine, plus the high phytate diet was enough cause for her osteomalacia.

11 There are two other causes for hip pain in this patient. At her age osteoarthritis is not uncommon, and the prolonged steroids may have caused aseptic necrosis of the femoral head. Referred pain from inflamed bowel in the pelvis, or from abscesses in or around the perineum, are other potential cause of hip pain.

Case 21

Arthritis and indigestion

A pleasant 72-year-old lady went to her primary-care physician complaining of severe pain in both her hips and knees. She had endured these symptoms for many years and they had progressively got worse, and the pain so intense that it made walking very difficult. She had not visited the doctor before as she did not want to waste his time. She had been trying to manage with paracetamol for pain relief but this was no longer effective. Her past history was of a hysterectomy for fibroids some 26 years earlier and a stomach ulcer treated by milk drip almost 50 years ago. The patient did not smoke and drank alcohol only on special occasions. On examination she was found to be overweight and had marked changes of osteoarthritis in both knees with marked crepitus, and some bony overgrowth. There was considerable restriction in joint movement both in the knees and to a lesser extent in both hips. She had marked Heberden's nodes in her hands.

Investigations

Haematology and Biochemistry chart on page 94. Radiology: osteoarthritis both knees (**1**).

1

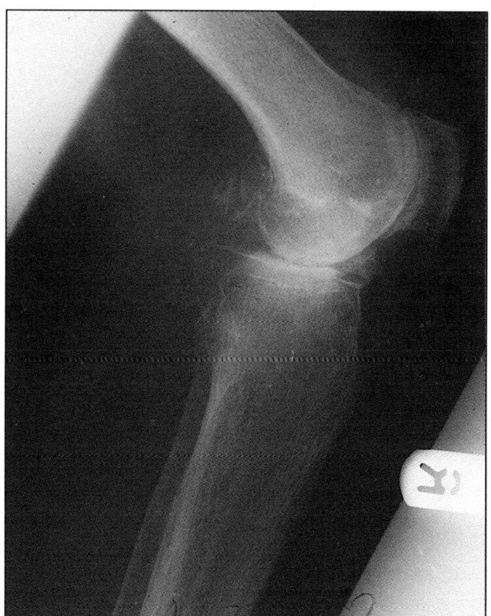

1 X-ray of the knee.

Question

1 What treatment would you prescribe for this patient?

		Normal Range			Normal Range
Hb	12.8	11.5–16.0 **g/dl**	**MCHC**	33.4	33–36 **g/dl**
Hct	38.3	33–47 **%**	**Platelets**	367	150–400/ **10^9/l**
MCV	85.6	80–100 **fl**	**WCC**	8.2	3.5–11 **/ 10^9/l**
MCH	28.6	28–33 **pg**	**ESR**	14	< 20 **mm/hr**
Sodium	144	135–145 **mmol/l**	**Blood sugar**	6.0	3.5–7.2 **mmol/l**
Potassium	4.9	3.5–5.0 **mmol/l**	**Bilirubin**	7	2–17 **mmol/l**
Chloride	100	95–105 **mmol/l**	**Alk. Phos.**	114	35–125 **U/l**
Bicarbonate	27	20–30 **mmol/l**	**ALT**	14	0–35 **U/l**
Urea	4.2	2.5–7.0 **mmol/l**	**GGT**	15	0–35 **U/l**
Creatinine	87	50–150 **mmol/l**	**Albumin**	47	36–52 **g/l**
Phosphate	1.39	0.7–1.4 **mmol/l**	**Globulin**	22	22–32 **g/l**
Calcium	2.34	2.2–2.6 **mmol/l**	**CRP**	<5	<5 **mg/l**

Answer and discussion

1 Initially analgesia alone would be the best choice with advice about weight reduction. Although osteoarthritis is not an inflammatory arthropathy, there is little doubt that non-steroidal anti -inflammatory drugs (NSAIDS) do give some relief to these patients. Ideally she should be referred to an orthopaedic surgeon for consideration of joint replacement.

Progress

The patient was started on NSAIDS and found that her mobility improved considerably. She had very little pain and was quite happy with her management. After a 5-month period, without warning she went to the toilet one morning and passed a large liquid black stool. She felt dizzy and sweaty and went back to bed after calling her doctor. When he arrived she was pale and clammy with a tachycardia of 120 beats per minute and a blood pressure of 100/60. He sent her into hospital by ambulance immediately.

Questions

2 What is the initial management of this patient?
3 What investigations would you organise?

Answers and discussion

2 Initial management involves the assessment of the cardiovascular state of the patient, as the need for resuscitation is the single most important decision that needs to be made. In this patient there was evidence of hypovolaemia with hypotension, tachycardia and signs of sympathetic overactivity. The prime aim must be to correct the haemodynamic state before proceeding to detailed investigation. It is obviously important for other causes, other than gastro-intestinal bleeding to be excluded. Thus a full examination is mandatory. If

there is no other cause found and melaena is confirmed on rectal examination, an intravenous infusion should be established, and while awaiting blood to be cross-matched a plasma expander may be used. Obviously, when blood is taken for cross-matching, samples can also be taken for full blood count and prothrombin time. It is also sensible in a patient of this age to check that her ECG is normal. Once blood is available, this should be given at a rate commensurate with her overall clinical condition. For very elderly patients, or those with cardiovascular, respiratory or renal disease consideration should be given to the insertion of a central venous line as these patients are at particular risk if over-transfused. Any patient seen with a significant gastrointestinal bleed should be managed by a joint gastroenterological/surgical team, and certainly those patients admitted with shock should be seen by a surgeon, in case the bleeding does not stop or the patient has a rebleed. The mortality from a rebleed is much greater than from the initial bleed. The overall mortality from gastrointestinal bleeding is around 10%. However, in those units that run a GI bleeding team or unit, the mortality can be reduced to less than 5%. The patient should thus, if possible, be admitted to an area of the hospital that specialises in the care of gastrointestinal bleeding and be monitored carefully.
3 After resuscitation, arrangements should be made for this patient to have the cause of the bleeding ascertained. The use of barium studies is no longer undertaken for this purpose in modern units and the investigation of choice to be organised is an oesophagogastroduodenoscopy. Her endoscopy is shown in **2**.

2

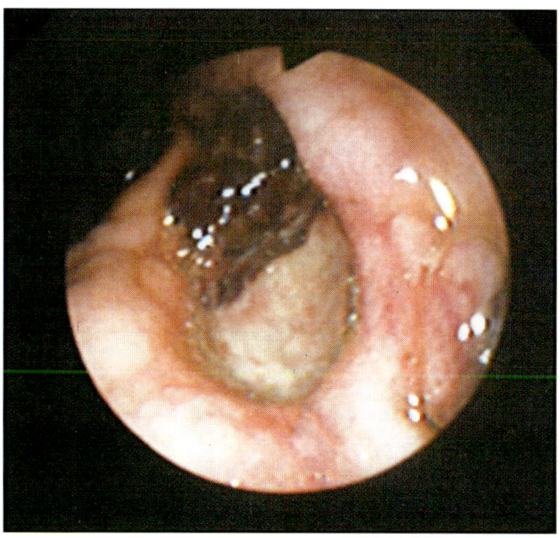

2 Endoscopy.

Questions

4 What does the endoscopy show ?
5 What are the indications for urgent upper gastrointestinal endoscopy?
6 What are the risks of emergency endoscopy ?
7 What are the indications for blood transfusion in a patient with an acute gastrointestinal bleed?
8 What treatment would you consider for this patient ?

Answers and discussion

4 The endoscopy shows an ulcer. The ulcer was high on the lesser curve and was difficult to see because of surrounding mucosal oedema.
5 The indications for urgent endoscopy are: if there is any suggestion that the patient might have oesophageal varices; if the patient has an underlying bleeding diathesis such as thrombocytopenia due to haematological disease ; if the bleeding continues and despite attempts at resuscitation, there is no improvement ; and if the patient has rebled. Ninety per cent of bleeds stop spontaneously; in many of the patients who have had no haemodynamic disturbance and have not needed transfusion, endoscopy can be left to the next day on a routine list. For those patients who have been shocked, or have required blood, it is probably sensible for them to be scoped as soon as possible once resuscitation is complete.
6 The risks of emergency endoscopy are greater than for a routine diagnostic endoscopy. First, the patient may not be fasting, or the stomach may be full of blood and thus the patient is at risk of aspiration on insertion of the endoscope. Second, if the patient is hypotensive and thus hypoxic, introduction of an endoscope into the oral cavity might increase the hypoxia and this will certainly be worse if the patient is given sedation. It is thus imperative that such patients are preoxygenated via nasal spectacles before endoscopy and that they are monitored carefully, preferably by pulse oximetry during the procedure. A further risk is more an organisational one. Many out of hours emergencies are dealt with by relatively inexperienced staff and for acute bleeders it is important that the endoscopy is performed by an experienced endoscopist with fully trained endoscopy assistants or endoscopy nurses and with proper equipment. Financial constraints often mean that this is rarely achieved. The final problem with emergency endoscopy is that in some the patient is bleeding so heavily that all that can be seen is blood, a so called 'red out'.
7 The indications for transfusion are an observed large haematemesis or melaena stool, signs of shock in association with a GI bleed, or a haemoglobin below 10g/dl.
8 The presence of a visible vessel in the base of an ulcer, an adherent clot or a black spot in an ulcer carries a greater than 50% chance of rebleeding. These findings are often referred to as Stigmata of Recent Haemorrhage (SRH). The mortality of a rebleed is higher than that of an initial bleed, and thus attempts to stop rebleeding are worthwhile considering. In ulcers without these stigmata or with oozing from the edge the rebleed rate is below 6%. There are two approaches to this problem. Either the patient can be offered early surgery, which has been shown in a series from Birmingham, UK to reduce the mortality by prevention of rebleeding. This policy will of course mean an increase in surgery with its attendent risks as well as operating on some patients (up to 50%) who would not have rebled anyway. The alternative is to use interventional endoscopic techniques to treat the vessel and prevent rebleeding. There are a variety of techniques that can be used, including injection therapy with noradrenaline, alcohol or sclerosants (**3**), the use of a diathermy probe (**4**), heater probe or laser treatment (**5**). All these techniques have been shown to be of benefit with perhaps the laser having the best results. Similarly these

3 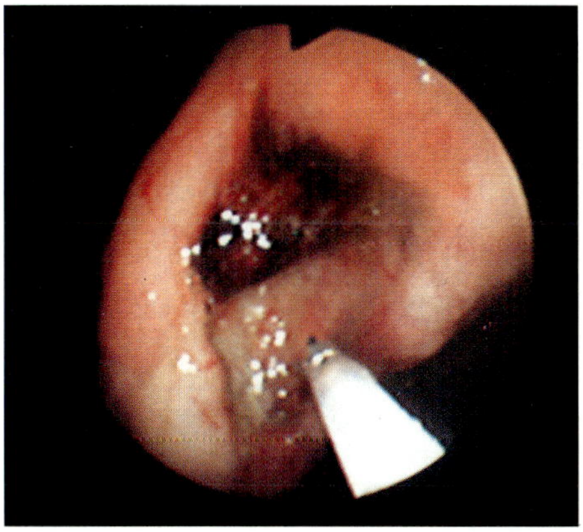 4
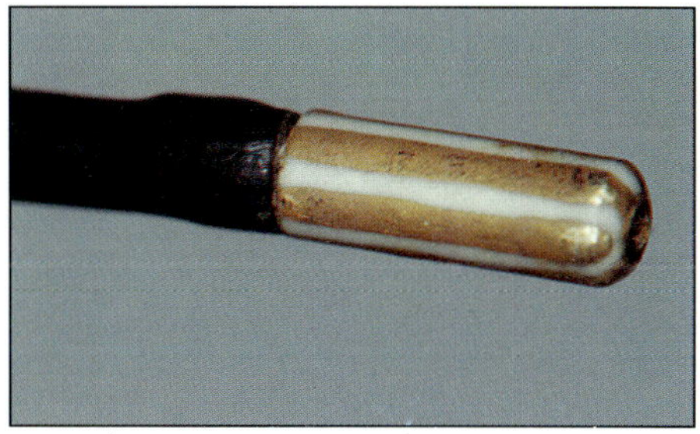

3 Injection of adrenaline into a gastric ulcer to stop bleeding.

4 Bicap diathermy probe tip.

5 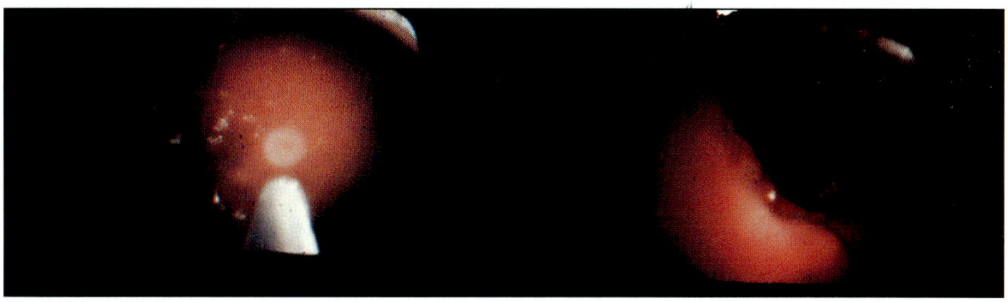

5 Positioning laser aiming beam on edge of ulcer crater.

techniques can be used to stop active bleeding, provided there is endoscopic access and a suitable lesion to treat. Endoscopic therapy in trained hands is simple to apply and rapid and adds very little to the time taken for the diagnostic endoscopy. Should it fail, the patient probably should have surgery, because second attempts at treatment increase the risks of perforation. Endoscopic therapy is ideal for unfit patients or those otherwise unsuitable for surgery. This patient had the ulcer lasered at the initial endoscopy; however, some 12 hours later she had a further massive bleed and her haemoglobin fell to 4g/dl. She was taken to theatre and the bleeding artery at the base of the ulcer was under-run with sutures. Because of her parlous state no acid reducing, anti-ulcer operation was undertaken. After appropriate blood replacement, the patient made a full recovery

Questions

9 What treatment would you now recommend for this patient ?
10 How would you prevent NSAID induced ulceration ?
11 What criticism could be made of her primary care physicians' management ?

Answers and discussion

9 This patient has thus had a bleed from a gastric ulcer that was presumably related to the ingestion of NSAIDS. It would thus be advisable for the NSAID to be stopped and the patient to be placed on a course of an ulcer-healing agent. Any ulcer-healing agent can be used, provided that it is given at full dose and for at least 2 months to ensure healing of the ulcer. All gastric ulcers should be examined at the end of a standard course of therapy to ensure full ulcer healing and to permit biopsy to exclude malignancy. There is now evidence that NSAID ulcers can heal, albeit more slowly, if the NSAID is continued. This has been shown clearly for ranitidine in studies of both NSAID induced duodenal and gastric ulcers. This patient was so frightened by her bleed that she refused to take any NSAID; however, after a few months her arthritis was so severe that she was both house-bound and at times wheelchair-bound. In desperation she requested advice as to how she could safely take NSAIDS.

10 There is no absolute guarantee that NSAID induced ulcers can be prevented in individual patients. Many drugs have been shown to have preventive effects, but there is no ideal therapy that meets the needs of simplicity, safety and efficacy. H_2 receptor antagonists have been shown to be effective at preventing duodenal ulceration, are simple to take and are remarkably safe. They do not, however, protect against gastric ulceration as effectively. Misoprostol, the prostaglandin analogue, is more effective at preventing against gastric ulceration than duodenal ulceration but has a higher side-effect profile and has to be taken at least twice a day. Proton pump inhibitors may be effective but have been subjected to less studies to date. Thus, to offer this patient maximum protection, it was decided to place her on long-term ranitidine and misoprostol. Once established on both of these, without side effects, the NSAID was reintroduced and the patient was gastroscoped at regular intervals to ensure there was no ulcer recurrence. It has been noted that many NSAID induced ulcers are silent. After 6 months of therapy, at repeat endoscopy, several small gastric erosions were noted (**6**). At this juncture the patient decided to come off the NSAID, even though life

6

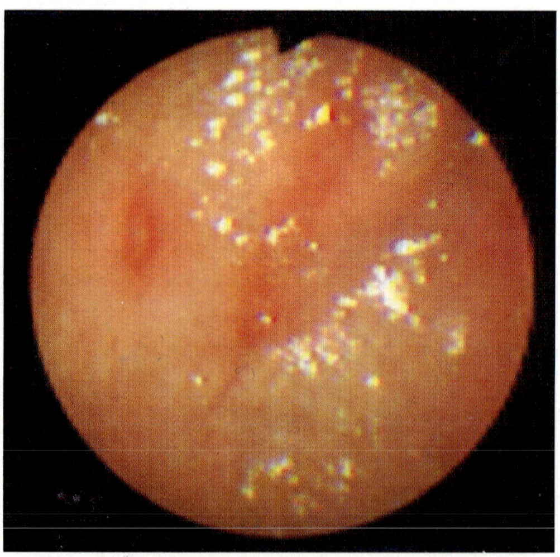

6 Repeat endoscopy after 6 months.

had been more tolerable. By this time her joints had deteriorated sufficiently for her orthopaedic surgeon to offer her joint replacement.

11 There is considerable debate as to whether all patients who are put on NSAIDS should receive routine ulcer prophylaxis at the same time. Many gastroenterologists would suggest that the elderly and infirm, infact those that would tolerate ulcer complications or the surgery for these complications poorly, should receive routine prophylaxis with either H_2 blockade or prostaglandin analogues. Another group of patients at risk are those patients with a history of previous peptic ulceration before starting NSAIDS. It has been shown that the ulceration rate in those patients with a previous history is five times greater than in those with no such history. Thus after 2 months of NSAID, up to 10% of patients will develop ulceration in their upper gastrointestinal tract, if there is no previous history of peptic ulceration, while in those with a previous history up to 50% will develop ulceration on NSAIDS in the same period. This group of patients is thus at major risk if started on NSAIDS and should always be protected. It is on this point that her primary care physician could be criticised. If there is a prior history of duodenal ulceration, an H_2 blocker should be co prescribed, if a gastric ulcer then a prostaglandin analogue.

Case 22

Dizziness and diarrhoea

This 28-year-old man presented at the accident and emergency department with a history of feeling generally unwell and being dizzy. The dizziness was postural and exertional and prevented him from playing football. For a couple of days before admission he had suffered mild diarrhoea and had started to vomit on the day of his admission. On examination he was a large man of athletic build. His pulse was 126 beats per minute with a lying blood pressure of 100/60 and a sitting blood pressure of 80/60 mm Hg. He had slight tenderness in his epigastrium, with normal bowel sounds. The bowl beside his bed contained definite coffee grounds, but on rectal examination there was no melaena.

Investigations

Haematology and Biochemistry chart on page 101.

Questions

1 How would you treat this patient?

Answers and discussion

1 Initial treatment should be aimed at correcting the signs of shock. An intravenous infusion should be started initially with a plasma expander until blood is cross-matched. This was done in this patient and he was transfused with 4 units of blood without any significant change in his condition. A repeat haemoglobin was measured and had risen to 15.8g/dl. A chest x-ray was normal and an ECG was performed (**1**).

1

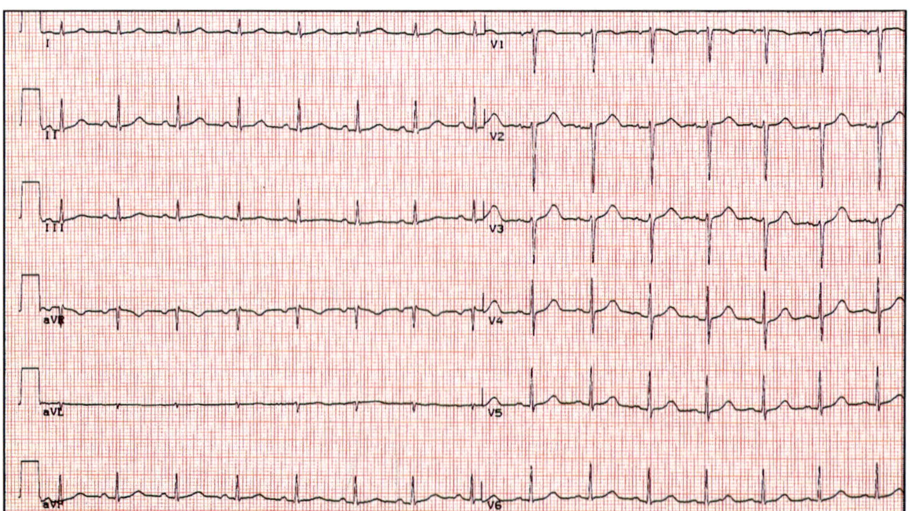

1 An ECG tracing of the patient.

		Normal Range			Normal Range
Hb	11.6	12.5–18 **g/dl**	**MCHC**	34.8	33–36 **g/dl**
Hct	36.4	33–47 **%**	**Platelets**	220	150–400/ **10^9/l**
MCV	85.0	80–100 **fl**	**WCC**	8.3	3.5–11 **/ 10^9/l**
MCH	29.6	28–33 **pg**	**ESR**	8	< 20 **mm/hr**
Sodium	126	135–145 **mmol/l**	**Blood sugar**	3.2	3.5–7.2 **mmol/l**
Potassium	5.9	3.5–5.0 **mmol/l**	**Bilirubin**	9	2–17 **mmol/l**
Chloride	96	95–105 **mmol/l**	**Alk. Phos.**	64	35–125 **U/l**
Bicarbonate	20	20–30 **mmol/l**	**ALT**	19	0–35 **U/l**
Urea	12.3	2.5–7.0 **mmol/l**	**GGT**	8	0–35 **U/l**
Creatinine	120	50–150 **mmol/l**	**Albumin**	37	36–52 **g/l**
Phosphate	2.35	0.7–1.4 **mmol/l**	**Globulin**	25	22–32 **g/l**
Calcium	3.8	2.2–2.6 **mmol/l**	**CRP**	<5	<5 **mg/l**

Questions

2 Is there a cause for his circulatory collapse seen on either his ECG?
3 What do the electrolyte results suggest is wrong?
4 What physical signs would you look for ?
5 How would you confirm the diagnosis ?
6 What treatment would you prescribe ?

Answers and discussion

2 The ECG is within normal limits and there is no obvious cause for his hypotension and tachycardia. There was thus a discrepancy between his physical signs and the response to transfusion. At this stage the junior doctors inserted a central venous line and confirmed that he had a low central venous pressure. Two further units of blood were given with no cardiovascular response but with a further rise in haemoglobin to 17.9 g/dl.

3 The electrolytes up to this time had been ignored. When all the results were reviewed in the light of his failure to respond, it was apparent that there were only two causes for his electrolyte disturbance. The patient was questioned as to whether he had taken any potassium sparing diuretics, to which there was a negative answer. It was at this point that the cause of his problem was diagnosed. Addison's disease or acute adrenal failure seemed to be the only reasonable diagnosis. The high urea had been attributed to his gastrointestinal bleed rather than to fluid depletion.

4 The patient was then re-examined to look for buccal pigmentation, pigmentation in his palmar creases or for any scars. No such changes were found. Figure **2** shows buccal pigmentation from another patient.

2

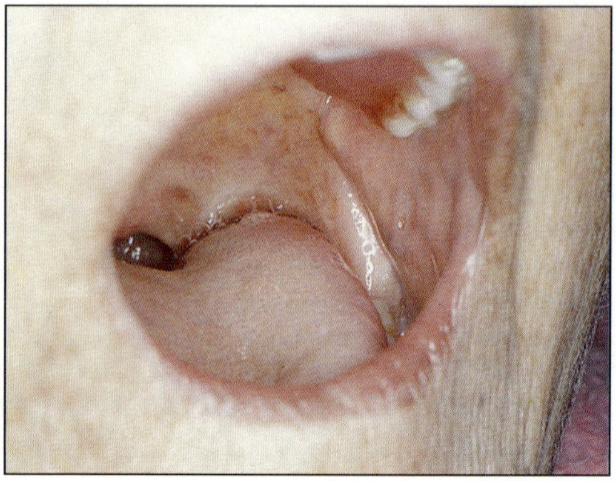

2 Buccal pigmentation in another patient.

5 A plasma cortisol level should be taken and an injection of ACTH given before a repeat cortisol half an hour later. Obviously in a shocked patient resuscitation takes precedence over completing the diagnostic tests, and adrenal stimulation tests were not performed at that stage. Instead, as well as a plasma cortisol, blood was taken for ACTH measurement. Neither test was available as an emergency and the blood was stored for later analysis. Eventually his cortisol result came back showing a very low level with an extremely high ACTH result, consistent with adrenal failure. An adrenal stimulation test was performed once the patient had recovered and with both a short (half hour) and long ACTH stimulation test there was no rise in cortisol or urinary steroids.

6 Once diagnosed, intravenous saline was given and intravenous hydrocortisone 100 mg. After a few hours, and 4 litres of normal saline, his blood pressure had risen to 120/75 lying with no postural drop. The following day he was feeling well and the intravenous fluids were discontinued. His intravenous hydrocortisone which had been given at a dose of 100 mg 6 hourly was discontinued and oral hydrocortisone substituted at a dose of 20 mg first thing in the morning and 10 mg in the afternoon. Fludrocortisone was also prescribed at a dose of 100 micrograms once daily. This regime kept him well and with normal electrolytes. The patient was given a card to carry with him at all times, which stated that he had Addison's disease. The next day endoscopy revealed mild antral gastritis.

This case stimulated a review of both patients with known adrenal failure and patients presenting with gastrointestinal emergencies. Vomiting, abdominal pain and diarrhoea are well recognised signs of adrenal failure, and indeed were often the presenting features of the disease. Admitting doctors should be aware of this and should think of this condition if the cardiovascular state is deranged out of proportion to the degree of gastrointestinal bleeding. Two weeks later an exactly similar case was diagnosed, this time without the administration of blood.

Case 23

Abdominal pain and alcohol

A 54-year-old joiner was referred to the clinic with a 6-month history of abdominal pain and back pain. In addition he had developed diarrhoea. He described the diarrhoea as being porridge like, pale and smelling strongly. He opened his bowels 3 times a day and there was never any history of rectal bleeding or passage of mucus. The abdominal pain had been constant and was sited in his epigastrium. In fact on closer questioning he had had bouts of abdominal pain for several years and the difference over the last 6 months was that the pain had been consistently present with no bouts of freedom. His previous bouts of pain usually had followed alcoholic binges and each bout had lasted for several weeks. He had been told he had gastritis but had never had any investigation. He was uncertain if the epigastric pain radiated through to the back, but there was always a constant pain in his back and to the left side of his chest posteriorly and up to his shoulder. He had noticed that he had lost a considerable amount of weight and was feeling tired and weak. He had always drunk large amounts of alcohol ever since he left school at 16 years of age. His current consumption was over 100 units per week, with him drinking up to 10 pints of beer per day. He smoked 40 cigarettes a day. On system review he complained of some thirst and frequency with regular nocturia 3 times a night. There was no dysuria or symptoms of prostatism. On examination he had marked pigmentation on his back (**1**). He was tender in his epigastrium but there was no mass palpable. His faeces are shown in **2**.

Investigations

Haematology and Biochemistry chart on page 104. Straight x-ray abdomen (**3**).

1

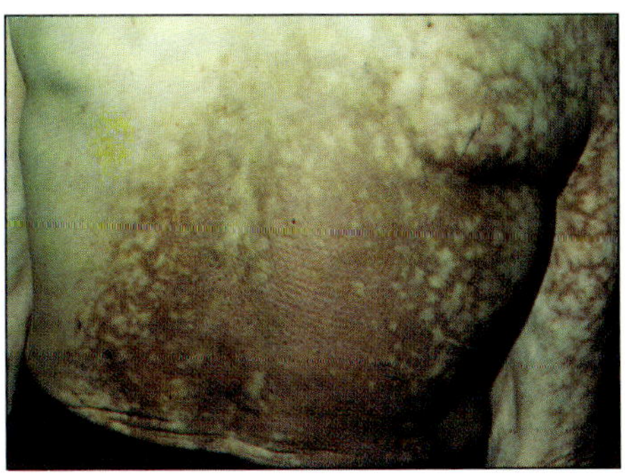

1 Pigmentation of the back.

2

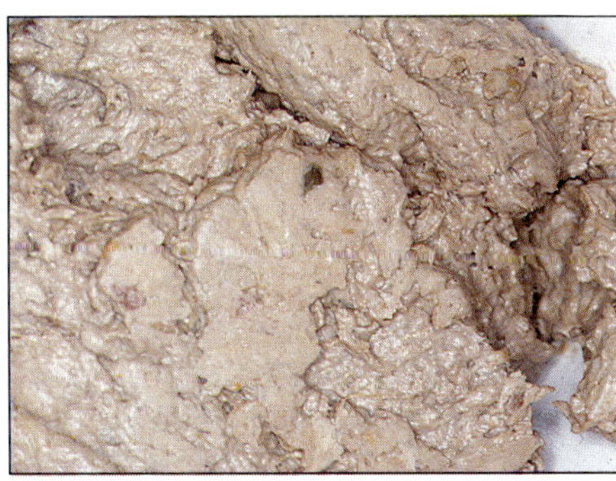

2 Patient's faeces.

Questions

1 What is the cause of the pigmentation on the back of the chest?
2 What does the abdominal x-ray show?
3 What is the full diagnosis?
4 How would you treat this patient?

3

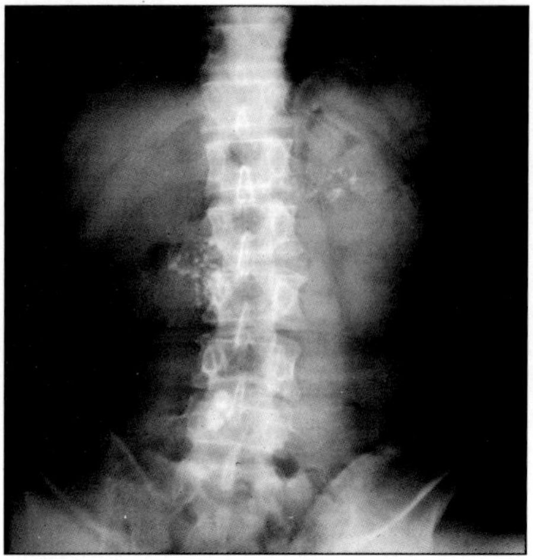

3 X-ray of the abdomen.

4

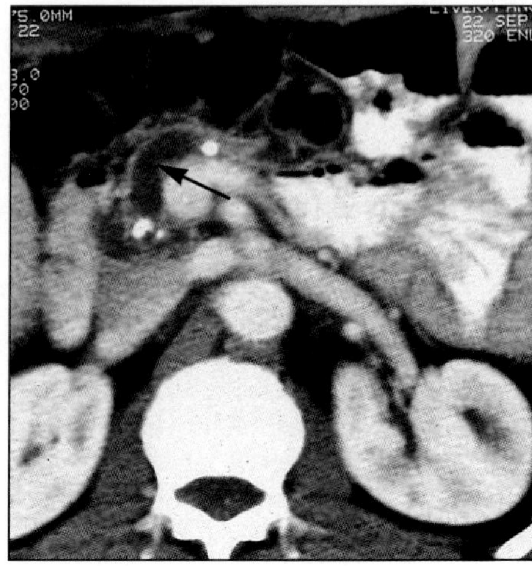

4 CT scan of the pancreas.

		Normal Range			Normal Range
Hb	12.6	12.5–18.0 **g/dl**	**MCHC**	34.6	33–36 **g/dl**
Hct	37.5	33–47 %	**Platelets**	163	150–400/ **10⁹/l**
MCV	105.8	80–100 **fl**	**WCC**	4.5	3.5–11 **/ 10⁹/l**
MCH	36.7	28–33 **pg**	**ESR**	7	< 20 **mm/hr**
Sodium	138	135–145 **mmol/l**	**Blood sugar**	12.7	3.5–7.2 **mmol/l**
Potassium	4.5	3.5–5.0 **mmol/l**	**Bilirubin**	14	2–17 **mmol/l**
Chloride	98	95–105 **mmol/l**	**Alk. Phos.**	162	35–125 **U/l**
Bicarbonate	29	20–30 **mmol/l**	**ALT**	35	0–35 **U/l**
Urea	4.2	2.5–7.0 **mmol/l**	**GGT**	104	0–35 **U/l**
Creatinine	60	50–150 **mmol/l**	**Albumin**	36	36–52 **g/l**
Phosphate	0.84	0.7–1.4 **mmol/l**	**Globulin**	25	22–32 **g/l**
Calcium	2.01	2.2–2.6 **mmol/l**	**CRP**	<5	<5 **mg/l**
Prothrombin time		18 **sec**	**Control**		13 **sec**

Answers and discussion

1 The pigmentation on the back is erythema ab igne due to the patient's habit of putting a hot water bottle on his back to try and get some pain relief.
2 The abdominal x-ray shows diffuse calcification in the area of the pancreas.
3 This patient has several interrelated diagnoses. He has:
a) Alcoholic chronic calcific pancreatitis
b) Diabetes mellitus
c) Malabsorption with prolonged prothrombin time and low calcium and marked steatorrhoea
d) Macrocytosis either due to the alcohol excess or malabsorption of folate or B_{12}
e) A raised GGT and Alkaline Phosphatase either due to alcoholic liver disease,

or to a degree of cholestasis from the chronic pancreatitis. The high alkaline phoshatase might be of bony origin and related to the low calcium.
4 Initially an assessment must be made as to whether the patient requires drying out with suitable drug cover to prevent withdrawal symptoms. The patient had no history of delirium tremens nor of morning craving and had never had any shakes. As he felt so unwell he was admitted and kept under close observation with instruction that should he develop any withdrawal symptoms or signs, he should be started on either chlormethiazole, diazepam or chlordiazepoxide to cover the withdrawal period. As far as his diabetes was concerned a blood sugar profile was performed over a 24-hour period and the results varied between 16 and 27 mmol/l. Oral hypoglycaemics failed to produce control and he was started on twice daily, self-administered insulin with good blood sugar control. Pain relief was obtained by use of regular paracetamol supplemented by dihydrocodeine. Some authorities believe that aspirin is effective at relieving the pain of chronic pancreatitis but this patient was unfortunately allergic to aspirin.

The management of the steatorrhoea involves checking that the patient is not consuming an excess of fat in his diet, and putting the patient on a restricted fat diet. With the dietary fat restriction, dietary advice should be sought from a dietitian working in conjunction with the local diabetologist. The amount of steatorrhoea can be reduced further by the prescription of pancreatic enzyme supplements to be taken with food. To preserve the action of these supplements either special delayed release formulations can be used to prevent inactivation of the enzymes by gastric acid or acid lowering drugs can be co -prescribed, such as a histamine $_2$ receptor antagonist or a proton pump inhibitor. Correction of any vitamin deficiencies is also of importance and in his case vitamin K and D supplements were administered. His folate and B_{12} levels were normal. Further investigation was undertaken and this confirmed gross steatorrhoea with a faecal fat of 24 gm/24 hours (normal less than 7 gm) A CT scan of his pancreas was undertaken (**4**). This shows pancreatic calcification and a distended pancreatic duct (arrow).

Progress

The patient abstained from alcohol for a couple of months but then started to drink again. He failed to attend clinic on several occasions but reported almost a year later with severe pain not controlled by pethidine prescribed by his general practitoner. An ERCP was undertaken after a repeat scan had shown no obvious change (**5**).

Questions

5 What does the ERCP show, and what was the indication for performing the test?
6 What are the contraindications to undertake an ERCP?
7 What forms of treatment are available for the relief of his pain?

Answers and discussion

5 The ERCP shows gross distortion of the pancreatic duct with clubbed side branches and several main duct strictures giving a beaded appearance to the duct. ERCP is indicated in chronic pancreatitis for several reasons. First, to assess the cause of jaundice and outline the biliary tree in those patients with cholestasis. Second, to determine the diagnosis of chronic pancreatitis in the

5

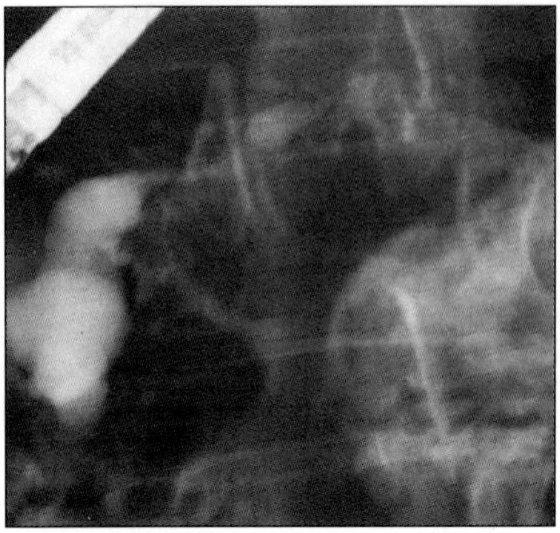

5 A repeat scan.

6

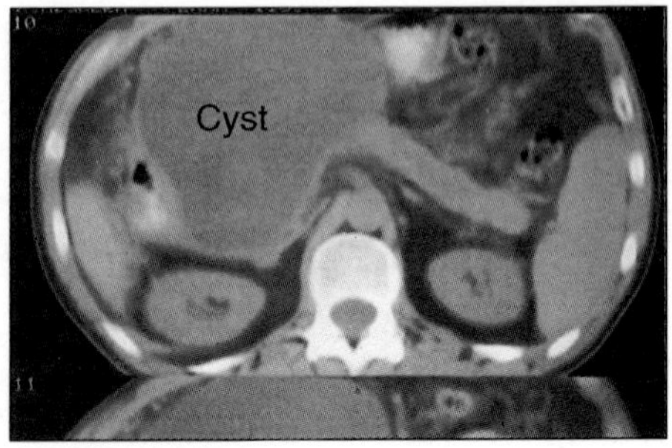

6 Pancreatogram.

absence of other features on x-ray or scanning. In some units pancreatic function tests are performed but in many the diagnosis is made on the basis of disordered structure as seen on scans, calcification on x-ray, or the typical appearance on pancreatography (ERP). The third main indication is to see if there is a remediable lesion in the pancreas, such as a localised stricture or stones in the pancreatic duct.

6 The main contraindication is the presence of a cyst or pseudocyst demonstrated in the pancreas on scanning. The risk is that of introducing infection into the cystic area and thus inducing a pancreatic abcess. ERP can be performed under these circumstances, if a surgeon is planning to go ahead with surgery shortly after the ERP, and needs the pancreatogram as a prerequisite of surgery. Allergy to contrast media, pyloric obstruction or duodenal obstruction in the second part are all relative contraindications, or factors that make ERP difficult as do duodenal diverticulae.

7 The mainstay of pain relief is the avoidance of alcohol. If the patient has abstained and the pain is only controllable by narcotic analgesics, then it is important to investigate to see if there is a treatable localised lesion. Recent developments in endoscopic therapy have been extended to include the balloon dilatation of strictures in the main pancreatic duct, stone removal from the pancreatic duct and even attempts at pancreatic ablation by injection of resin into or tissue glue into the duct to sclerose the whole duct. Only the techniques of balloon dilatation and stone removal have been widely practised and offer some help. Stent insertion through a pancreatic duct stricture is generally confined to malignant strictures.

If the disease is diffuse and without a localised treatable abnormality, then the option lies between resection of the pancreas by a skilled surgeon or referral to a pain-relief specialist for consideration of a coeliac-plexus block.

If a pseudocyst is present, either percutaneous needle aspiration drainage or surgical drainage will often relieve the pain. Figure **6** shows a large cyst, that drained percutaneously. If the cyst is in communication with the pancreatic duct, percutaneous drainage may result in pancreatic fistula. This patient stopped drinking, remaining abstinent for over 12 months. His pain gradually settled and was controllable by simple analgesics.

Case 24

Dysphagia and diarrhoea

This 38-year-old lady presented with a 2-month history of heartburn, pain on swallowing and a 1-month history of dysphagia. The dysphagia was predominantly for solids but was not particularly progressive. She had lost some weight but otherwise felt quite well. Haematology and Biochemistry chart on page 108.

Questions

1 What treatment would you give to this patient?
2 What initial investigations would be appropriate?

Answers and discussion

1 Dysphagia and odynophagia are symptoms that should always be taken seriously. Odynophagia, or pain on swallowing usually signifies ulceration or inflammation in the oesophagus. Although it would be permissible to prescribe something for the heartburn, such as antacids or a histamine_2 receptor antagonist, this should only be done while investigation is being organised. Dysphagia should be thought of as a sinister symptom together with weight loss, bleeding or anaemia and severe vomiting. These symptoms must be investigated at presentation, and not after a trial of some medicament or other.

2 It is important in the investigation of dysphagia to exclude any physical obstruction such as a tumour or peptic stricture. The choice of investigation is between a barium swallow and an endoscopy. It used to be common practice to initiate investigation with a barium x-ray, but either is acceptable. There are advantages to both techniques and frequently both are required for full assessment. Endoscopy permits biopsy and therapy to be performed but is not as good as a barium study at demonstrating motility or length of a stricture (unless dilatation is undertaken at the first endoscopy).This patient had a barium swallow (**1**) organised by her primary care physician. When the patient was seen in the outpatient department, it was noticed that the skin of her hands was abnormal (**2**).

1

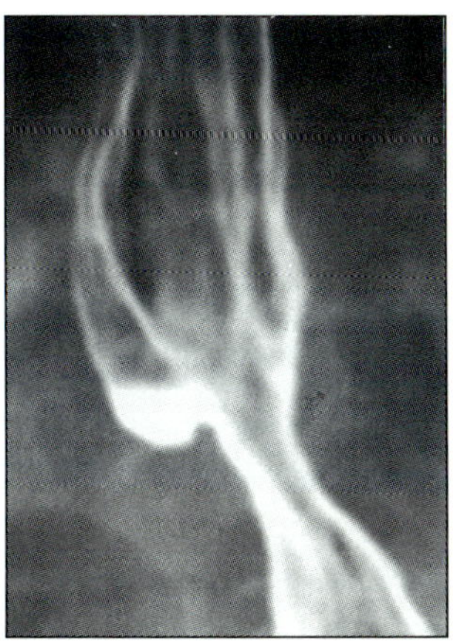

1 Barium swallow.

2

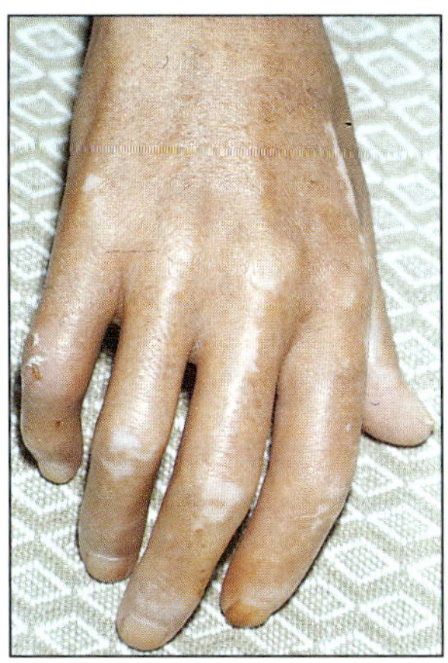

2 Abnormal skin.

3

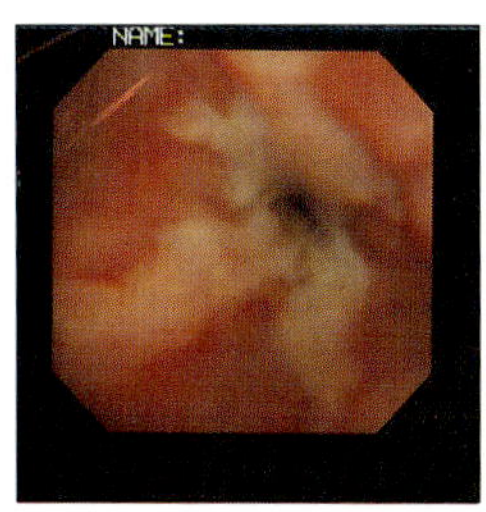

3 Endoscopic view.

Questions

3 What does the x-ray show?
4 What is the skin lesion?
5 What other questions would you ask this patient?
6 How would you treat this patient?

		Normal Range			Normal Range
Hb	10.6	11.5–16.0 **g/dl**	**MCHC**	28	33–36 **g/dl**
Hct	33	33–47 %	**Platelets**	210	150–400/ **10^9/l**
MCV	82	80–100 **fl**	**WCC**	5.6	3.5–11 **/ 10^9/l**
MCH	26	28–33 **pg**	**ESR**	12	< 20 **mm/hr**
Sodium	139	135–145 **mmol/l**	**Blood sugar**	3.2	3.5–7.2 **mmol/l**
Potassium	4.4	3.5–5.0 **mmol/l**	**Bilirubin**	9	2–17 **mmol/l**
Chloride	104	95–105 **mmol/l**	**Alk. Phos.**	58	35–125 **U/l**
Bicarbonate	25	20–30 **mmol/l**	**ALT**	6	0–35 **U/l**
Urea	52	2.5–7.0 **mmol/l**	**GGT**	12	0–35 **U/l**
Creatinine	88	50–150 **mmol/l**	**Albumin**	34	36–52 **g/l**
Phosphate	1.04	0.7–1.4 **mmol/l**	**Globulin**	30	22–32 **g/l**
Calcium	2.27	2.2–2.6 **mmol/l**	**CRP**	<5	<5 **mg/l**

Answers and discussion

3 The x-ray shows a stricture in the lower oesophagus which is smooth and has no shoulders. The appearances are of a benign peptic stricture. Endoscopy was undertaken to confirm the nature of the stricture and to biopsy it, as well as to undertake oesophageal dilatation. Figure **3** shows the endoscopic appearances with marked ulceration and stricture formation, while **4** shows some of the range of dilators that are available.

4 The hands show the changes of advanced scleroderma. There is thickening of the skin with areas of pigmentation and depigmentation. Surprisingly the patient had not mentioned the skin changes to her doctor, even though they were now interfering with her life such that she was having difficulty manipulating small objects. Figure **5** shows her face with smoothing of the skin and decrease in size of her mouth, due to the sclerodermatous process. She had recently found that she could not sing properly in her church choir.

5 In any patient with dysphagia, it is important to ask if they suffer from Raynaud's phenomena, particularly if there is no abnormality seen on endoscopy or radiology. In the absence of an obstructing mass lesion, the association of Raynaud's with dysphagia should make you think of scleroderma or systemic sclerosis. In the presence of sclerodermatous changes, the history of Raynaud's and dysphagia suggests the CREST syndrome. It would thus be appropriate to

4 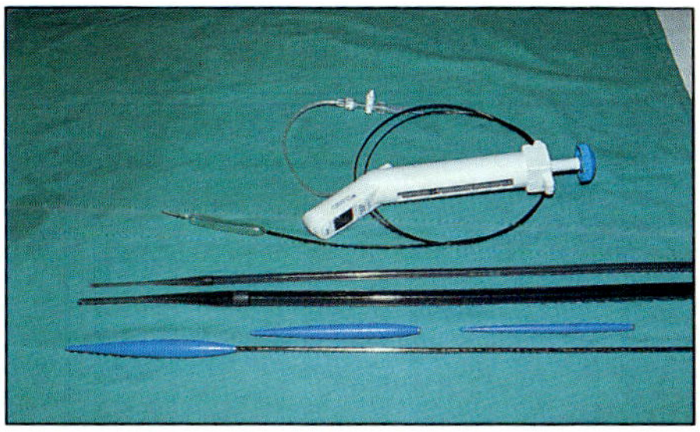

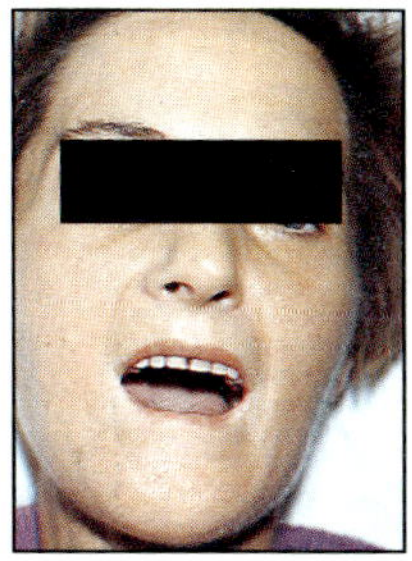 5

4 Range of dilators.
5 Note skin and size of mouth.

look for the other signs of this syndrome — telangiectasia and calcinosis.
6 Treatment should be aimed at relieving the dysphagia and heartburn, helping her cope with her disability and consideration of treatment of her underlying disease. Peptic oesophagitis is treated by dilatation and acid suppression. Many gastroenterologists would prescribe a proton pump inhibitor for the severe grades of oesophagitis. Dilatation is performed when required and the frequency usually reduces with time. To cope with the increasing disability various aids are required, such as large-handled cutlery, gadgets to pick things up from the floor, and the help of an occupational therapist is indicated to fully assess the patient's needs. There is unfortunately no cure for systemic sclerosis or scleroderma. However, trials of Cyclosporin A have shown some benefit in a few patients. Not all patients with the CREST syndrome have oesophagitis or stricture formation as a cause for their dysphagia and some have free reflux demonstrated on their x-ray. These patients should be placed on prophylactic acid suppression to try and prevent the development of oesophagitis and stricturing. Remember that oesophagitis alone can cause dysphagia without the presence of stricturing. In the absence of any oesophagitis or stricture, the next investigation would be an oesophageal manometry study. Several months later the patient reattended clinic complaining of diarrhoea, which was foul smelling and difficult to flush. A breath hydrogen test with dextrose was undertaken and the result is shown in **7**, and a barium follow through (**8**) was performed.

Questions

7 What does the manometry (**6**) study show?
8 What are the possible causes of the diarrhoea?
9 What do the breath hydrogen and small bowel x-ray show?
10 How would you treat this patient?

Answers and discussion

7 The motility study shows no peristalsis with weak amplitude swallow induced waves, which are not propagated down the length of the oesophagus. This is a typical finding in systemic sclerosis.
8 The most likely cause of diarrhoea in a patient with advanced systemic sclerosis is bacterial overgrowth caused by a 'blind loop syndrome' secondary to impaired small-bowel motility. Of course other causes of diarrhoea are possible and it must not be assumed that this is the underlying cause. Investigation must therefore be aimed at demonstrating both evidence of bacterial overgrowth as well as of impaired small-bowel motility.
9 The breath hydrogen test shows a large early rise in hydrogen level consistent

6 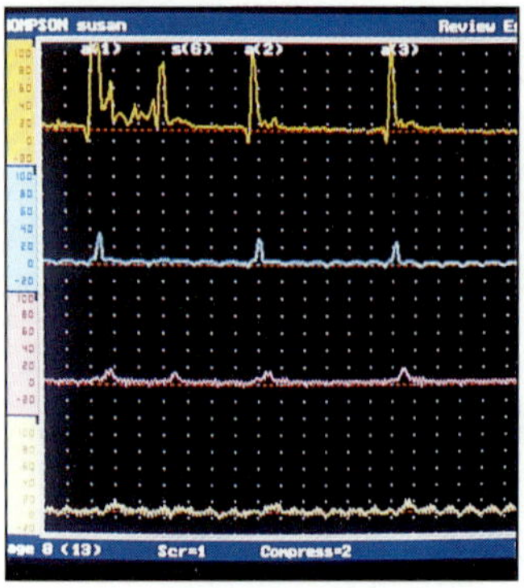

8 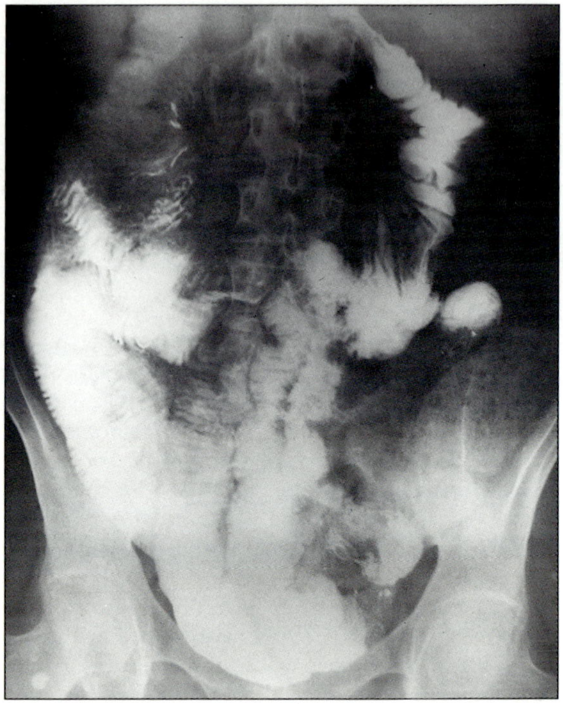

7

Time	Hydrogen concentration
8.30	0 - 5
	0 - 5
	0 - 5
8.35	75g Dextrose
8.40	10
8.45	19
8.50	27
8.55	31
9.10	55
9.25	69
9.40	70
9.55	73
10.25	63
10.55	44
11.10	38
11.25	32

6 Manometry study.

8 Barium follow through.

7 Hydrogen test.

with bacterial overgrowth. Some centres use a C^{14} glycine cholate breath test instead or as well as the breath hydrogen test. Few use small-bowel intubation and aspiration and culture of jejunal fluid, partly because of the difficulty in intubation and also because of the difficulty in culturing the samples under both aerobic and anaerobic conditions.The barium follow through shows grossly dilated loops of small bowel with oedematous folds (producing the so-called 'stacked coined' appearance. The barium took many hours to traverse the small intestine, confirming the delayed transit and providing the ideal conditions of stasis and stagnation for bacterial overgrowth.

10 A course of antibiotics is the treatment of choice usually initially with oxytetracycline 250–500 mg three times daily. If this fails to work, a common second choice is to use metronidazole 200-400 mg three times a day. After a few weeks course it is sensible to stop treatment if it has been effective, to see how long it takes for symptoms to return. If rapid return of symptoms occurs, long-term treatment with either a single antibiotic, or with alternating courses of antibiotics may be required. If relapse is long delayed, then intermittent courses are all that is required and patients should be given a course of tablets to keep at home. Some patients do not improve and they may require combinations of antibiotics or other types of antibiotic. Failure to respond should signify investigation of other causes of diarrhoea and malabsorption.

Case 25

Postoperative diarrhoea

This pleasant 64-year-old ex-paratrooper was referred with a history of disabling diarrhoea ever since having an operation for an ulcer. About 8 years previously he had developed typical symptoms of a duodenal ulcer, with nocturnal epigastric pain that would wake him at night, post prandial pain that came on 30 minutes after eating and was relieved by antacids. His primary care physician had referred him to a local general surgeon who had arranged a barium meal. This showed a duodenal ulcer (**1**). He had been given a course of cimetidine for 1 month which had completely removed his symptoms; however, they returned some 8 weeks later while on holiday in Rome and he was started on a second course by the hotel doctor. On returning to the UK he attended for a follow-up appointment with the surgeon who advised him that he needed an operation. He was not warned of any potential side effects and after some persuasion agreed to surgery. He had his operation and within a few days of the operation noticed that his stools were looser. He was told that he had had his gall bladder removed as well as having the main nerves to his stomach cut. The surgeon told him that his gall bladder was full of stones. Over the next year his diarrhoea got progressively worse so that he found he could no longer work as a security guard. He had extreme urgency, such that if he could not find a toilet immediately he was incontinent. Eventually the only way he could go out in his car was by having a portable toilet in the boot of his car (**2**). Apart from being prescribed codeine and loperamide, he had been offered little help. Eventually he demanded a second opinion. On examination there was nothing to find except his midline epigastric scar.

Investigations

Haematology and Biochemistry chart on page 112; Endoscopy(**3**).

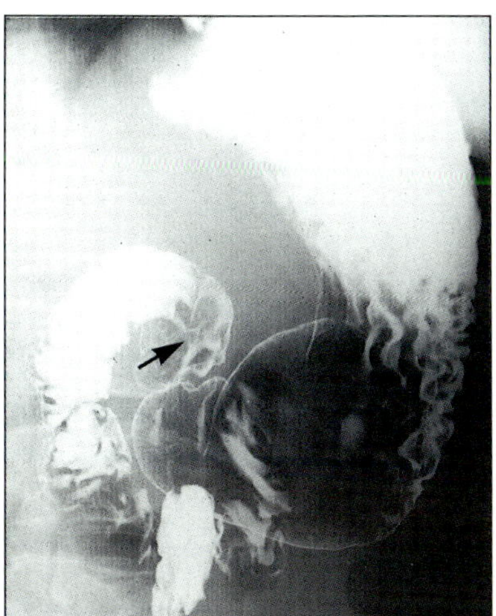

1 Barium meal showing duodenal ulcer (arrow).

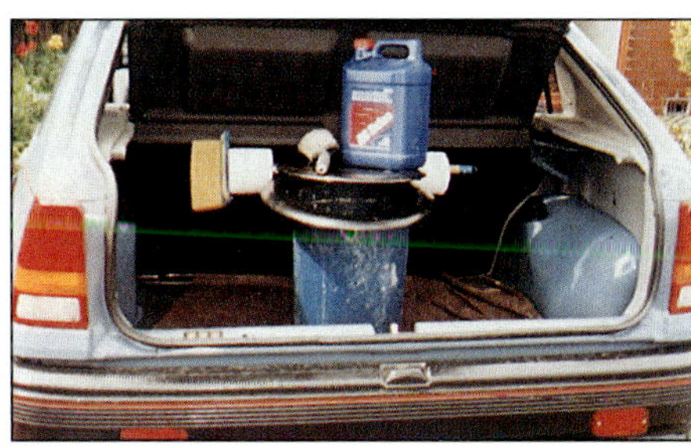

2 Portable toilet in boot of car.

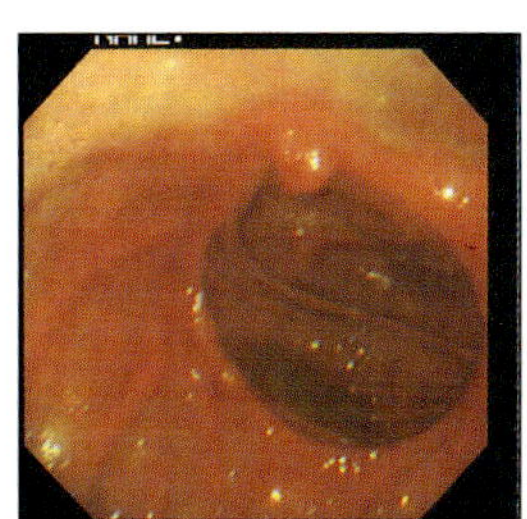

3 Gastroscopy.

Case 25

Questions

1 What does the gastroscopy (**3**) show?
2 What are the possible causes of his diarrhoea?
3 what further investigations would you undertake?

		Normal Range			Normal Range
Hb	11.6	12.5–18.0 **g/dl**	**MCHC**	34.8	33–36 **g/dl**
Hct	36.4	33–47 %	**Platelets**	220	150–400/ **10^9/l**
MCV	85.0	80–100 **fl**	**WCC**	8.3	3.5–11 **/ 10^9/l**
MCH	29.6	28–33 **pg**	**ESR**	8	< 20 **mm/hr**
Sodium	126	135–145 **mmol/l**	**Blood sugar**	9	3.5–7.2 **mmol/l**
Potassium	5.9	3.5–5.0 **mmol/l**	**Bilirubin**	64	2–17 **mmol/l**
Chloride	96	95–105 **mmol/l**	**Alk. Phos.**	19	35–125 **U/l**
Bicarbonate	20	20–30 **mmol/l**	**ALT**	8	0–35 **U/l**
Urea	12.3	2.5–7.0 **mmol/l**	**GGT**	50	0–35 **U/l**
Creatinine	120	50–150 **mmol/l**	**Albumin**	25	36–52 **g/l**
Phosphate	2.35	0.7–1.4 **mmol/l**	**Globulin**	<30	22–32 **g/l**
Calcium	3.8	2.2–2.6 **mmol/l**	**CRP**	<5	<5 **mg/l**

Answers and discussion

1 The gastroscopy shows a gastroenterostomy. The surgeon had performed a vagotomy and gastroenterostomy and on looking through the operative notes it was not clear why this rather than a pyloroplasty had been performed. There was no suggestion at operation of pyloric stenosis or marked scarring which might have precluded a pyloroplasty.

2 There are many potential causes for post-gastric surgery diarrhoea. Many doctors ascribe the diarrhoea to being simply due to the truncal vagotomy. This undoubtedly does occur, but usually comes on immediately after the operation and is not progressive. The frequency of such diarrhoea has been quoted as from 10–20%, a figure that rises if the patient also has a cholecystectomy. This is thought to result from the constant passage of bile salts into the bowel in association with intestinal hurry due to the vagotomy. It is particularly difficult to treat. The fact that this patient's diarrhoea got worse with time suggests there may be other mechanisms involved. The diarrhoea may be due to unmasking of some latent bowel disease such as coeliac disease, although this is rare. Simple intestinal hurry due to the gastroenterostomy remains as one cause and is often associated with symptoms of dumping. Bacterial overgrowth due to the gastroenterostomy and the reduction in acid secretion consequent upon the vagotomy is another cause. A form of choloretic diarrhoea can also occur due to the rapid transit with increased ileal loss of bile salts into the colon and the associated bile salt induced (choloretic) diarrhoea.

3 Initial investigation should be aimed at determining if there is any specific mechanism of diarrhoea that can be treated before trying simple constipating agents. Thus a gastric emptying study will determine how quickly food leaves the stomach, and a small-bowel biopsy will exclude coeliac disease. To exclude bacterial overgrowth either small-bowel aspiration and culture, breath hydrogen or labelled C^{14} glycine cholate breath test can be used. To test for the possibility of choloretic diarrhoea a gamma labelled bile salt can be given and its retention in the body measured. Selenium labelled Homo-Cholic-Acid-Taurine, (SeHCAT) is a labelled artificial bile acid conjugated to taurine. It should not be forgotten that other causes of diarrhoea may occur unrelated to the operation, such as lactose intolerance, small-bowel Crohn's disease or colonic diseases.This patient had a normal small-bowel biopsy and went on to have a radionucleide gastric emptying study (**4**), breath hydrogen test (**5**) and SeHCAT study.

Questions

4 What do the studies in **4** and **5** demonstrate?
5 What treatment would you give to this patient ?

4

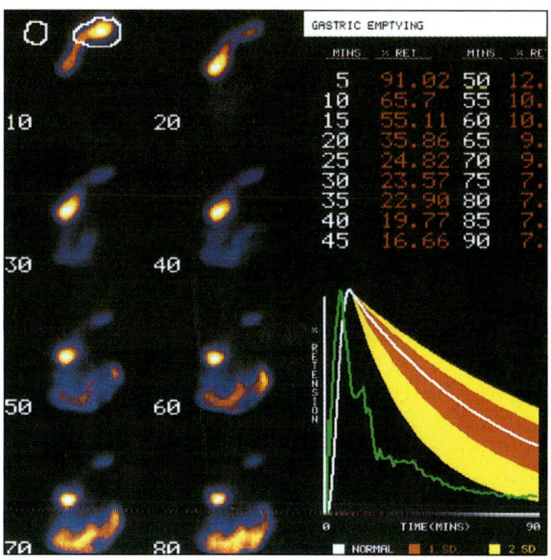

4 Radionucleide study of gastric emptying.

Answers and discussion

4 The gastric emptying study shows rapid gastric emptying in comparison with the normal range. This matched the observed rapid gastric emptying seen on a barium examination where most of the barium was seen to go through the gastroenterostomy. Barium is of course not physiological and transit measurements with barium do not necessarily correlate with more physiological measurements. Isotope gastric emptying studies use labelled food and thus more closely resemble normal circumstances. In the study shown the meal consisted of a sandwich containing radioactively labelled

5
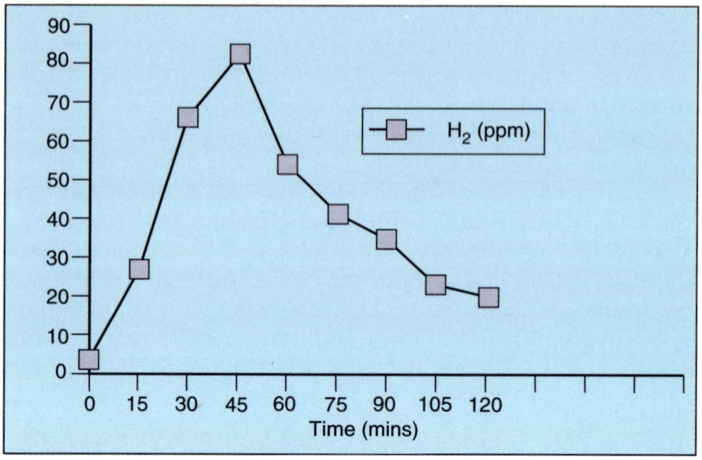

5 Study of dextrose breath test.

bran as well as a drink. This is used as a solid phase marker. The breath hydrogen test demonstrates an early significant rise in hydrogen levels consistent with bacterial overgrowth. There is, however, the possibility that because of the rapid transit through the gastroenterostomy the substrate used for the breath hydrogen test (dextrose) might reach the colon before it is fully absorbed and thus give rise to an early peak. In view of the very early rise in hydrogen levels this was thought to be unlikely. The SeHCAT test showed that only 5% of the administered dose is still in the patient at 1 week, whereas under normal circumstances more than 16% should be present. This indicates significant loss of labelled bile salt, which is thought to equilibrate with the endogenous bile salt pool, thus indicating excessive loss from the circulating bile salt pool. It is implied that the excess loss into the colon and hence out of the body will on its way cause a choloretic diarrhoea.

5 From thc above investigations there appears to be at least three possible mechanisms for the diarrhoea without having to implicate the vagotomy, which may of course cause diarrhoea, but which is not in itself specifically treatable.

Bacterial overgrowth can be treated by either oxytetracycline 250–500 mg 3 times a day, or by metronidazole 200–400 mg 3 times a day. On oxytetracycline this patients diarrhoea reduced considerably such that he was no longer incontinent; however, he still had significant frequency of defaecation with loose stools. It was decided to try him on a bile-salt binding agent (cholestyramine), which further reduced his stool volume and increased the thickness of his motions to a toothpaste like consistency. The patient was delighted with this treatment and was able to discard his portable toilet in the car and get out without fear of urgency and incontinence.

The third possible form of treatment is aimed at reducing the rate of gastric emptying. Conventionally this is undertaken by using drugs that slow intestinal transit, such as codeine-based preparations or loperamide. These had already failed in this patient. If no other mechanism can be found for the diarrhoea, and there is no significant pyloric obstruction, then taking down of the gastro-enterostomy can help such patients. Even with minor degrees of pyloric narrowing, dilatation of the pylorus may offer the opportunity for revisionary surgery. Ante-peristaltic loops of small bowel have not proved to be of much help in difficult cases of true post vagotomy diarrhoea.

Questions

6 What other complications can result from very rapid gastric emptying following gastric surgery?
7 What other complications of gastric surgery for peptic ulceration can occur?

Answers and discussion

6 Rapid gastric emptying can give rise to either early or late dumping. Early dumping is thought to be due to the rapid emptying of a hyperosmolar load from the stomach into the small bowel with rapid indrawing of fluid into the bowel lumen to try to attain iso-osmotic conditions. This flow of fluid into the bowel results in depletion of the intravascular fluid compartment with consequent dizziness and faintness. There is some evidence that part of the early dumping syndrome is due to small bowel distension and release of vasoactive humoral substances. The late form of dumping occurs when the rapidly emptying gastric contents stimulates an excessive release of insulin due to the very rapid increase in blood sugar. The insulin secretion may be excessive due to enteroglucagon release and sensitisation of the islet cells. The patient feels dizzy, light-headed and may become pale and sweaty, and in severe cases can even become confused and drowsy. The investigation of dumping syndrome is not particularly difficult. After the demonstration of rapid emptying a prolonged glucose tolerance test should be undertaken with bloods taken every quarter of an hour for both blood sugar and packed cell volume. Figures **6** and **7** show the typical blood sugar and packed cell volume results in patients with early and late dumping. The volume effects can be

6

Time (mins)	Packed cell volume (%)	Blood glucose (mmol/l)	Symptoms
0	47.0	4.6	Nil
0	46.8	4.1	Nil
Dextrose 75mg			
15	46.5	9.8	Abdominal discomfort
30	45.4	10.1	Feeling of fullness
45	45.3	9.7	Fullness / Nausea / Weakness
60	43.7	8.3	Abdo. symptoms resolving
75	43.1	6.7	Weak / Tremulous
90	45.3	6.6	
105	46.2	6.2	Symptoms resolving
120	46.3	5.6	
135	45.9	5.3	Attack over
150	46.8	5.8	
165	46.6	4.9	
180	46.9	4.8	

6 Early dumping.

7

Time (mins)	Packed cell volume (%)	Blood glucose (mmol/l)	Symptoms
0	42.7	5.4	Nil
0	42.5	5.9	Nil
Dextrose 75mg			
15	43.0	7.2	
30	42.6	6.1	
45	41.8	6.9	
60	41.7	5.7	
75	41.7	5.5	
90	42.0	4.5	
105	41.4	3.2	Hunger
120	40.6	1.6	Tremulous / weak
135	42.1	1.4	Sweaty / tremulous/ weak
150	43.0	2.1	Weak
165	42.2	3.8	Symptoms beginning to resolve
180	42.8	3.6	

7 Late dumping.

limited by taking small dry meals with low sugar content and with fluids taken separately. The hypoglycaemia can be controlled in some by restricting the sugar and carbohydrate content of meals, in others by using guar gum to try and delay absorption, but in the difficult case by use of preprandial subcutaneous injections of octreotide (a somatostatin analogue).

7 The complications of peptic ulcer surgery depend in part upon the type of operation performed. Highly selective vagotomy has fewer side effects and complications than the more traditional forms of peptic ulcer surgery. Malabsorption with resulting anaemia and other forms of anaemia are relatively common after gastric resections. Post- gastrectomy bloating, biliary gastritis and alkaline reflux oesophagitis are other complications. There is now good evidence that 15–20 years after partial gastric resection there is an increase in gastric carcinoma arising in the gastric remnant. Recurrent ulceration can occur after any form of gastric surgery and is least after vagotomy and antrectomy. The recurrent ulceration rate with highly selective vagotomy depends on the expertise of the surgeon.

Case 26

Doctor with diarrhoea

A 53-year-old female general practitioner requested a consultation because of altered bowel habit. She had previously had good health and had normally opened her bowels 1–2 times per day with a soft formed stool. For about 4 months she had noticed some looseness of her motions that had become porridge like in consistency. She had noted the passage of some mucus for a similar length of time but had passed no blood until the day before she had contacted the gastroenterology department. During the 4 months she had noticed some abdominal distension towards the end of each day, and had rectal dissatisfaction. She had also noted mild colicky left iliac fossa pain which was relieved by defaecation for the preceding 3 weeks. She had been under a lot of stress in her practice and felt that her symptoms got worse when the stress was particularly bad. There was no other relevant history and her appetite was normal and weight constant. Both parents had developed bowel cancer in their 70s and she was anxious about her symptoms. On examination there was no abnormality in the abdomen and rectal examination was normal.

Investigations

Haematology and Biochemistry chart on page 118. Sigmoidoscopy (**1**)

Questions

1 What is the likely diagnosis ?
2 What further investigation should be undertaken ?
3 What is the relevance of the finding shown in **1** ?

1

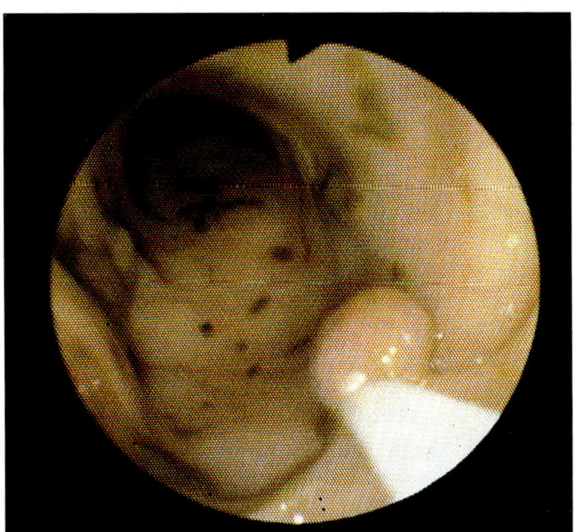

1 Small polyp being removed using a snare.

		Normal Range			Normal Range
Hb	13.1	11.5–16.0 **g/dl**	**MCHC**	34.3	33–36 **g/dl**
Hct	38.0	33–47 **%**	**Platelets**	239	150–400/ **10^9/l**
MCV	87.2	80–100 **fl**	**WCC**	7.4	3.5–11 **/ 10^9/l**
MCH	30.0	28–33 **pg**	**ESR**	12	< 20 **mm/hr**
Sodium	137	135–145 **mmol/l**	**Blood sugar**	4.8	3.5–7.2 **mmol/l**
Potassium	3.9	3.5–5.0 **mmol/l**	**Bilirubin**	4	2–17 **mmol/l**
Chloride	104	95–105 **mmol/l**	**Alk. Phos.**	75	35–125 **U/l**
Bicarbonate	27	20–30 **mmol/l**	**ALT**	13	0–35 **U/l**
Urea	3.1	2.5–7.0 **mmol/l**	**GGT**	21	0–35 **U/l**
Creatinine	64	50–150 **mmol/l**	**Albumin**	45	36–52 **g/l**
Phosphate	1.17	0.7–1.4 **mmol/l**	**Globulin**	32	22–32 **g/l**
Calcium	2.20	2.2–2.6 **mmol/l**	**CRP**	<5	<5 **mg/l**

Answers and discussion

1 The most likely diagnosis would have been an irritable bowel syndrome (IBS), if it had not been for the passage of blood. Patients with rectal bleeding should not be labelled as an IBS case until a cause for the bleeding has been determined. There are several types of IBS – the constipation and pain predominant type, the alternating diarrhoea and constipation type, the painless diarrhoea predominant type and the bloated patient.

2 Investigation of IBS should always include a sigmoidoscopy, but what further investigation is undertaken will depend upon the individual patient. In the young patient with a typical history further investigation may not be warranted, unless there are atypical features or the patient demands reassurance. For atypical symptoms, or in those patients presenting for the first time over the age of 40 it is probably wise to undertake some further investigation such as barium enema or colonoscopy. In this particular patient the presence of rectal bleeding alone should indicate the need for more detailed colonic investigation. In most centres colonoscopy is the investigation of choice for rectal bleeding, and in this patient the presence of the small polyp and the family history should make colonoscopy mandatory.

3 The tiny polyp shown in **1** is unlikely to be the cause of this patient's symptoms, except for the passage of blood. It has, however, got a greater significance in that it indicates the need for full assessment of the colon to ensure there are no other polyps higher in the colon. Her positive family history alone is enough to indicate the need for further colonic investigation. Colonoscopy also allowed the removal of the polyp by snare polypectomy. The rest of this patient's colon was normal at colonoscopy, with no other polyps and only a few sigmoid diverticulae.

Questions

4 What are the common precipitants or aetiological factors in IBS ?
5 What treatment would you advise ?

Answers and discussion

4 Stress is one of the most commonly blamed precipitants of IBS. This may or may not be accompanied by depressive features. Food intolerances are said by some to be a common cause and must be clearly distinguished from true, immunological type food allergy, which is rarely implicated. Many female patients seem to present to gastroenterologists after gynaecological procedures or operations. It is not always clear whether their original symptoms were actually gynaecological or simply a form of IBS. Most commonly the presenting symptom was suprapubic pain with distension, often exacerbated before or during menstrual periods. This is frequently due to hormonal effects on smooth muscle in the bowel making the symptoms worse. Post infective IBS following an acute gastrointestinal infection or food poisoning is also well recognised, as is IBS following multiple courses of antibiotics. The latter may result from alterations in normal gut flora. There is no doubt that in some patients no underlying cause or precipitating factors can be found. Many studies have shown electromyographic and transit abnormalities in patients with IBS; however, the cause of these changes is unknown.
5 In this patient an essential part of the treatment was the reassurance the negative colonoscopy gave her. In view of the family history and the small adenomatous polyp found, she was entered into the polyp-surveillance programme. A repeat colonoscopy was performed after 1 year which was clear and she was then entered into a 3-yearly colonoscopy programme. This will be continued to the age of 75. From the point of view of her IBS symptoms, after firm reassurance her symptoms continued and the pain became a nuisance. Antispasmodics in the form of peppermint-oil capsules completely relieved the pain. The only problem that did not improve was the altered bowel habit, which gradually changed so that she was passing 5–6 watery motions per day. She found this very inconvenient as it interfered with her practice. Bulking agents had no effect and constipating drugs such as codeine and loperamide caused a recurrence of her pain. It was decided to try her on an exclusion diet to see if she had any food intolerances. It was quickly found that with the reintroduction of milk her diarrhoea returned.

Questions

6 What further basic investigations would you perform ?
7 Figures **2a** and **2b** shows two breath hydrogen curves. Which do you think belongs to this patient ?
8 What other investigations are required ?
9 What are the causes of this disorder ?

Answers and discussion

6 In view of the response to the introduction of milk either a lactose -tolerance test using blood-sugar measurements in response to an oral load of lactose or a lactose breath test should be performed. The latter does not involve taking blood and has replaced the lactose-tolerance test in many centres. The principle

2a

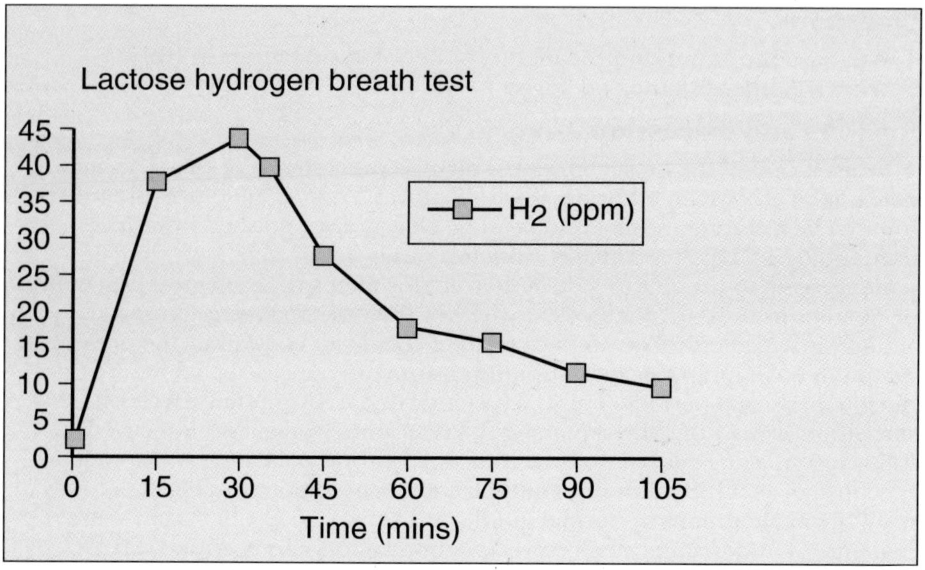

2a and **2b** Two hydrogen breath tests.

2b

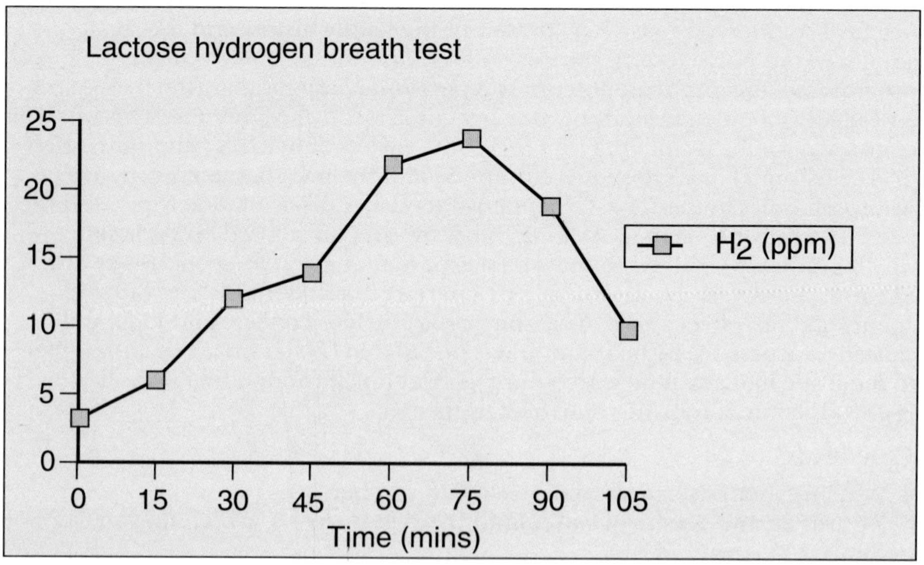

involves the ingestion of lactose, which in normal subjects is split by microvillal lactase and is absorbed as glucose and galactose. In patients with lactase deficiency, the lactose cannot be split and thus remains within the bowel lumen where it is osmotically active. Therefore, the lactose draws fluid into the bowel lumen and gives rise to an osmotic diarrhoea. The sugar-rich solution flows into the colon where the bacteria split the sugar and generate hydrogen. This diffuses across the bowel wall to reach equilibrium with the blood and is carried to the alveolae in the lung, where the hydrogen again diffuses across the lung to reach equilibrium with the alveolar air. This is then measured by an electrogenic hydrogen sensitive cell to produce a reading in parts per million.

7 The two breath hydrogen curves both show a rise in hydrogen levels in the end expiratory air during the course of the studies. Curve A shows an immediate rise in hydrogen, which is more characteristic of bacterial overgrowth in the upper small bowel or of a high jejuno-colic fistula. Curve B, which is this patient's curve, shows a rise occurring 30 minutes after ingestion of the lactose, which is consistent with the hurry associated with the osmotic diarrhoea.

8 As lactose intolerance has been demonstrated, it is important to ascertain if there is underlying small-bowel disease. A jejunal biopsy was performed and is shown in **3**. This shows subtotal villous atrophy consistent with coeliac disease. Had the biopsy been normal in some units, samples of the small-bowel mucosa would be assayed for lactase levels.

3

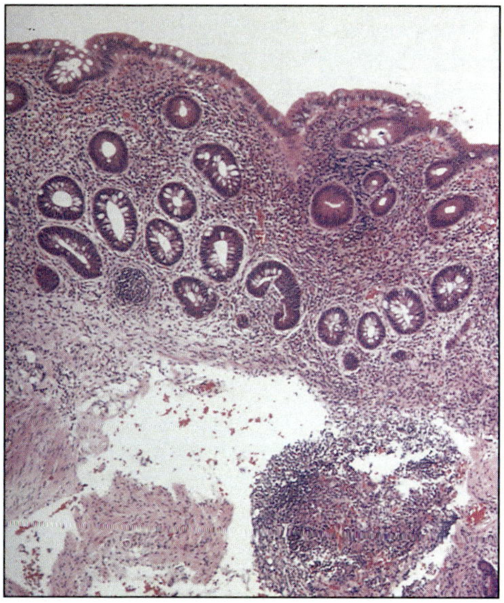

3 Segment from a jejunal biopsy.

9 The commonest form of lactose intolerance is the racially determined type, where the enzyme lactase is found in reduced concentrations in Asians, Chinese and Africans. The two other common varieties are the post infective temporary lactose intolerance often seen after gastroenteritis in children, and the lactose intolerance secondary to the reduced levels of enzyme secondary to causes of villus atrophy. The commonest of these in the West is coeliac disease. Rarely, some babies are born either with an absence of the lactase enzyme or with an inactive enzyme.

Case 27

Haematemesis and melaena

This 57-year-old man presented with a history of recurrent bouts of haematemesis and melaena. He had endured four such attacks in a period of 18 months, but none had been bad enough to require transfusion. Investigation at his local hospital had been negative on each occasion. He had four upper gastrointestinal endoscopies and the only finding on one occasion was a small amount of altered blood in the duodenum and antrum without a mucosal abnormality. During his last two attacks he had been found to have abnormal liver function tests, but the referring doctors were certain that he did not have varices within the range of the standard endoscope. He was referred for more detailed studies with the possibility of small-bowel enteroscopy. In his past history he had had rheumatic fever as a child and had mixed aortic and mitral-valve disease. He had been in atrial fibrillation for many years and 4 years previously had infective endocarditis following dental treatment with inadequate prophylaxis. From the cardiovascular point of view he had minimal symptoms and was able to work as a clerk. He had exertional dyspnoea on climbing stairs. His medication was warfarin, digoxin and a mild diuretic.

On transfer to our unit he was well and slightly icteric. His atrial fibrillation was well controlled and he had no signs of cardiac failure. He had the murmurs of mitral regurgitation and aortic stenosis. There were no signs of either chronic liver disease or infective endocarditis.

Investigations

Haematology and Biochemistry chart on page 123.

Questions

1 What are the causes of failure to find the source of upper gastrointestinal bleeding ?
2 What other symptom would you question the patient about ?
3 What are the possible causes of this patients symptoms ?
4 What further investigations would you undertake ?

Answers and discussion

1 The common causes of failure to identify the site of bleeding are:
a) The lesion is missed, usually due to obscuring blood or food or occasionally to delay in performing the endoscopy with healing of minor lesions.
b) The abnormal area has not been considered, such as bleeding from the retronasal space, pharynx or even tonsils.
c) The lesion has not been reached as in low duodenal or jejunal lesions, or in bleeding from the pancreas or biliary tract.
d) The bleeding is factitious.

About 10% of upper gastrointestinal bleeds do not have a cause identified, at least on the first occasion. The referring doctor had looked carefully in the pharynx and had always performed the endoscopy within 24 hours of the patient presenting. His view had not been obscured on any occasion.

		Normal Range			Normal Range
Hb	14.2	12.5–18.0 **g/dl**	**MCHC**	34.2	33–36 **g/dl**
Hct	41.6	33–47 %	**Platelets**	339	150–400/ **10^9/l**
MCV	94.5	80–100 **fl**	**WCC**	5.8	3.5–11 **/ 10^9/l**
MCH	32.4	28–33 **pg**	**ESR**	4	< 20 **mm/hr**
Sodium	140	135–145 **mmol/l**	**Blood sugar**	3.9	3.5–7.2 **mmol/l**
Potassium	3.8	3.5–5.0 **mmol/l**	**Bilirubin**	10	2–17 **mmol/l**
Chloride	101	95–105 **mmol/l**	**Alk. Phos.**	122	35–125 **U/l**
Bicarbonate	27	20–30 **mmol/l**	**ALT**	12	0–35 **U/l**
Urea	3.7	2.5–7.0 **mmol/l**	**GGT**	16	0–35 **U/l**
Creatinine	97	50–150 **mmol/l**	**Albumin**	38	36–52 **g/l**
Phosphate	0.74	0.7–1.4 **mmol/l**	**Globulin**	22	22–32 **g/l**
Calcium	2.23	2.2–2.6 **mmol/l**	**CRP**	<5	<5 **mg/l**
Prothrombin time		38 **sec**	**Control**		12 **sec**

2 This patient had upper gastrointestinal bleeding and unexplained jaundice. The presence of abdominal pain in association with the haematemesis would complete the classical triad associated with haemobilia. The patient was questioned carefully about this and did complain of upper right quadrant pain after his last haematemesis, which he had put down to the effort of vomiting. The pain had not been severe.

3 The triad of symptoms of upper GI bleed, jaundice and abdominal pain usually signifies bleeding from within the liver or biliary tree. This usually results from an arteriobiliary fistula and the pain is thought to be due to clot colic in the biliary tree. Melaena is more common than haematemesis. The common causes of this rare syndrome are from tumours within the liver or biliary tract. Less commonly stones may cause bleeding by erosion into the mucosa. False aneurysms, following trauma to the liver and after liver biopsy are relatively common, while in the Far East ascaris is a common cause. True aneurysms are seen in patients with polyarteritis nodosa and after infective endocarditis.

4 If there is a clear history of haemobilia, then arteriography would be the investigation of choice. Scanning to look for a mass lesion may help, particularly if there has been liver injury as a haematoma may be obvious. In patients from developing countries and the Far and Middle East, ascariasis must be considered and an ERCP would then be the most relevant investigation. In the absence of abnormal liver function tests, a small-bowel enteroscopy to look further down the gastrointestinal tract would be appropriate. It is not uncommon for patients on oral anticoagulants to bleed from their gastrointestinal tracts, particularly if their control is not good and the prothrombin ratio is kept at the upper limit of the therapeutic range or exceeds it.

Progress

The patient underwent arteriography and the angiogram is shown in **1**.

Questions

5 What does the angiogram demonstrate?
6 How would you treat this lesion?

1

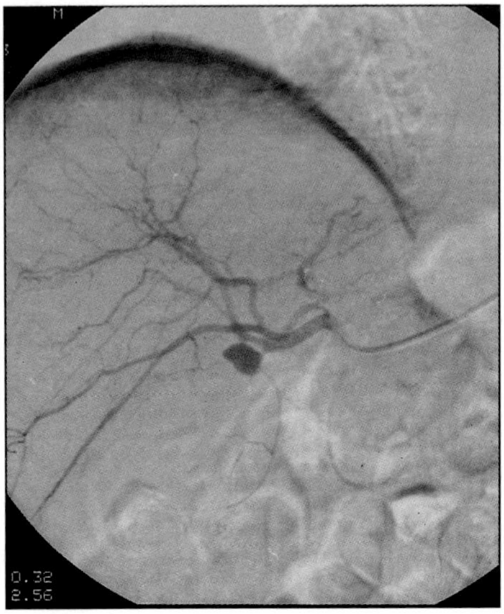

1 Angiogram.

2

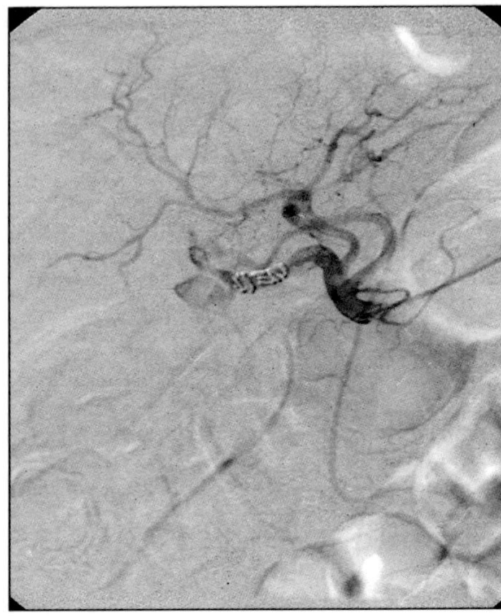

2 Arteriogram.

Answers and discussion

5 The angiogram shows a hepatic artery aneurysm, which was thought to be the result of his previous infective endocarditis. The diagnosis was thus a mycotic aneurysm of the hepatic artery.
6 The best initial form of treatment would be to embolise the artery at the time of the arteriogram. This was performed in this patient as is shown in **2**. The patient had no further problems on follow-up for 3 years. If embolisation was not feasible for technical reasons, then hepatic artery ligation would be one option or even segmental hepatic resection.

Case 28

'Bloody diarrhoea'

A 24-year-old student was referred with a history of recurrent episodes of anaemia responsive to iron therapy over the preceding 8 years. This had never been investigated fully until her present episode. There was no history of bowel dysfunction, overt bleeding nor symptoms of malabsorption. Her periods were slightly heavier than usual, and had been for a couple of years. However, a gynaecologist had examined her recently and found nothing wrong. On examination there were no physical signs to suggest a cause for her anaemia, and in particular there were no telangiectatic spots seen.

Investigations

Haematology and Biochemistry chart on page 126.

Questions

1 What are the common causes of this type of anaemia in young women?
2 How would you investigate this patient initially ?

Answers and discussion

1 There are two main groups of causes a) obstetric and gynaecological and b) gastroenterological. This patient had not had any children and despite some history of menorrhagia had no obvious gynaecological abnormality. From the gastroenterological point of view iron deficiency anaemia is either due to malabsorption or to blood loss. The commonest causes of malabsorption in the west are coeliac disease and Crohn's disease. At her age the common causes of blood loss are either from peptic ulceration or colonic polyps or inflammation. Tumours are uncommon at this age in comparison with patients over the age of 40 presenting with anaemia.
2 Initial investigations should include an upper gastrointestinal endoscopy with duodenal biopsies, thereby excluding any cause for bleeding in the upper GI tract as well as coeliac disease. It is always worth taking duodenal biopsies in patients with unexplained anaemia, because anaemia is frequently the only manifestation of coeliac disease. If these tests are normal, then in the presence of positive faecal occult blood tests, a colonoscopy would be the next investigation. A barium enema is not bad at excluding large mass lesions and moderately severe changes of colitis but is less good at demonstrating small polyps and minor colitic changes or vascular lesions. If all these tests are negative, then small-bowel radiology would be the next investigation, or in those units with the facilities, small-bowel enteroscopy. She had all the above tests performed with no abnormality seen. She decided against further investigation as the time off for her investigations was interfering with her course work. About 6 months before her final exams she made an urgent appointment, because she had developed 'bloody diarrhoea'. When she came to the clinic, on questioning she had actually been passing dark red liquid stools for several days and was feeling tired and light-headed. Her haemoglobin had dropped to 5.8 g/dl. She was admitted and transfused.

Question

3 What further investigation would you undertake?

		Normal Range			Normal Range
Hb	9.8	11.5–16.0 **g/dl**	**MCHC**	31.9	33–36 **g/dl**
Hct	30.7	33–47 **%**	**Platelets**	371	150–400/ 10^9/l
MCV	76.1	80–100 **fl**	**WCC**	7.1	3.5–11 / 10^9/l
MCH	24.3	28–33 **pg**	**ESR**		< 20 **mm/hr**
Sodium	144	135–145 **mmol/l**	**Blood sugar**	3.9	3.5–7.2 **mmol/l**
Potassium	4.3	3.5–5.0 **mmol/l**	**Bilirubin**	5	2–17 **mmol/l**
Chloride	100	95–105 **mmol/l**	**Alk. Phos.**	85	35–125 **U/l**
Bicarbonate	24	20–30 **mmol/l**	**ALT**	12	0–35 **U/l**
Urea	5.8	2.5–7.0 **mmol/l**	**GGT**	15	0–35 **U/l**
Creatinine	67	50–150 **mmol/l**	**Albumin**	48	36–52 **g/l**
Phosphate	0.80	0.7–1.4 **mmol/l**	**Globulin**	27	22–32 **g/l**
Calcium	2.50	2.2–2.6 **mmol/l**	**CRP**	<5	<5 **mg/l**
Serum iron		4.8 **µmol/l** (13–32)	**TIBC**	71 **mmol/l** (45–70)	
Serum transferrin		3.95 **g/l** (2.2–4)	**Saturation**	7%	
			Ferritin	6 **µg/l** (17–165)	

Answer and discussion

3 If the patient is actively bleeding on admission and is passing either melaena or dark red blood per rectum, it is sensible to repeat the gastroscopy as lesions can be missed on the first occasion. This was done in this patient and no abnormality was seen. Because the endoscopy was negative, and while she was being transfused mesenteric arteriography was undertaken. This should be performed by an experienced radiologist with good equipment, to be able to maximise the effectiveness. Her angiogram is shown (**1**).

Questions

4 What does the angiogram show?
5 Why might the angiogram fail to show a lesion?
6 What do the other angiograms show in **2–4**?
7 What further investigation is worth considering in this patient?

Answers and discussion

4 The angiogram shown is normal with no evidence of active bleeding, nor of any tumour blush or abnormal blood vessels.
5 The commonest reason for not seeing a lesion is that very commonly the patient has stopped bleeding even though they are still passing blood per rectum. Other reasons are technical difficulties in selectively catheterising some vessels, and that the lesion is too small for the technique to delineate.
6 Figure **2** shows a tumour blush in the jejunum of a patient while **3** shows typical colonic angiodysplasia (arrow).

7 In young patients with obscure GI bleeding, it is sensible to exclude a Meckel's Diverticulum. Although this is sometimes seen on small bowel radiology (**5**) this can not be relied upon. A Technetium isotope scan may be of value in the detection of ectopic gastric mucosa. On the basis of this, a laparotomy was performed at which a broad-necked Meckel's diverticulum was found and removed. The patient made a rapid recovery, has had no further bleeding, and her anaemia has not returned.

1

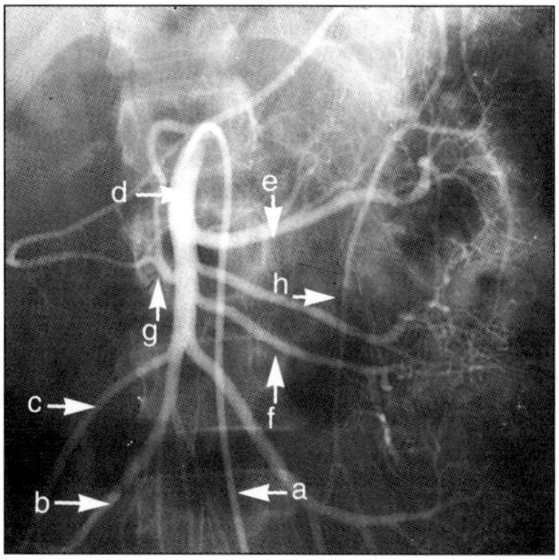

2

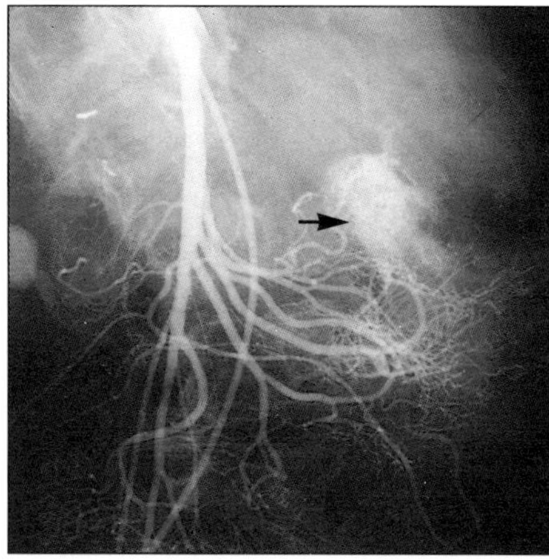

1 Arteriogram: **a** angiography catheter, **b** ileocolic artery, **c** right colic artery, **d** superior mesenteric artery, **e** jejunal artery, **f** ileal artery, **g** mid colic artery, **h** marginal artery.
2 and **3** Angiograms.
4 Another angiogram of colonic angiodysplasia showing early venous drainage. The other features are early mesenteric filling and vascular lakes.
5 Radiograph showing Meckel's Diverticulum of the small bowel.

3

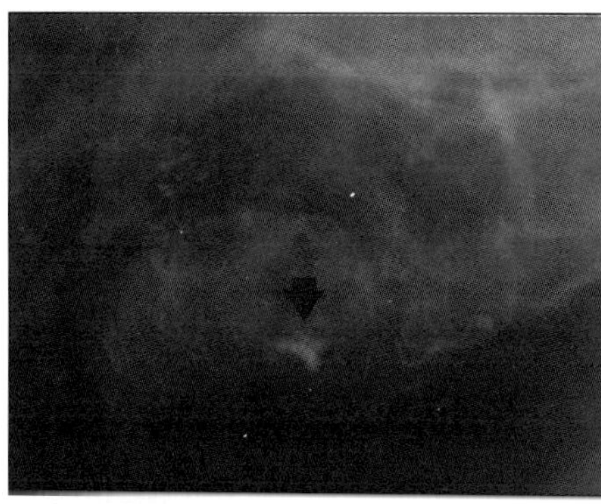

4

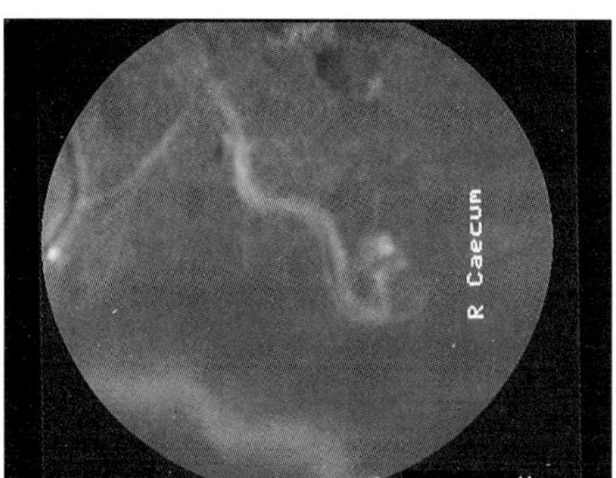

5

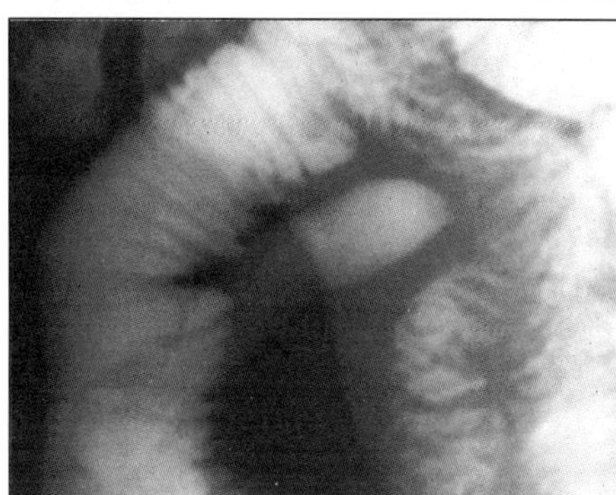

Index